Depression –
a nurse's experience

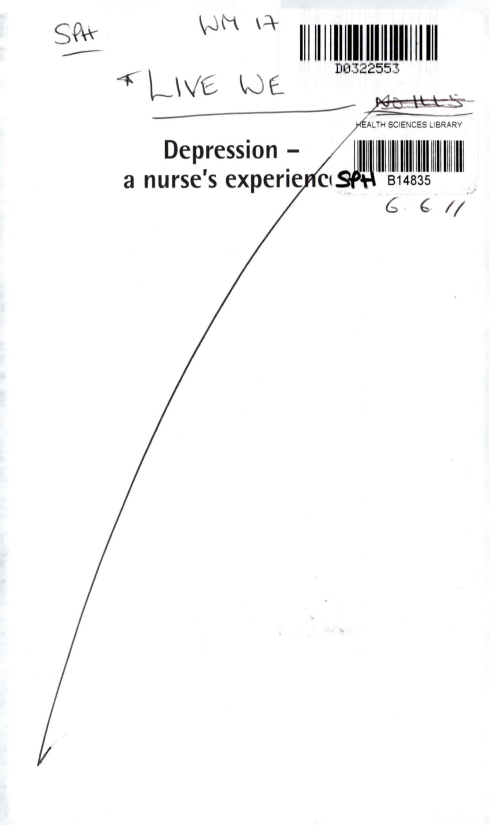

Depression –
a nurse's experience
shadows of life

VERONICA BURTON

Foreword by
PAUL FARMER
Chief Executive, Mind

Radcliffe Publishing
Oxford • New York

Radcliffe Publishing Ltd
18 Marcham Road
Abingdon
Oxon OX14 1AA
United Kingdom

www.radcliffe-oxford.com

Electronic catalogue and worldwide online ordering facility.

British Library Cataloguing in Publication Data

A catalogue record for this book is available from the British Library.

ISBN-13: 978 184619 305 7

The paper used for the text pages of this
book is FSC certified. FSC (The Forest
Stewardship Council) is an international
network to promote responsible
management of the world's forests.

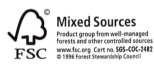

Mixed Sources
Product group from well-managed
forests and other controlled sources
www.fsc.org Cert no. SGS-COC-2482
© 1996 Forest Stewardship Council

Typeset by Pindar NZ, Auckland, New Zealand
Printed and bound by TJI Digital, Padstow, Cornwall, UK

Contents

Foreword

As a society, we are still beginning to come to terms with mental health as an issue. Despite the fact that one in four of us will experience a mental health problem in our lifetime, it remains misunderstood. We know that most people who experience mental health problems face stigma and discrimination in their daily lives – discrimination which may be from friends or family or in the workplace.

However, slowly but surely attitudes are changing. The *Time to Change* campaign, led by Mind and Rethink, is reaching large numbers of people with a simple message that we can all help tackle the stigma and discrimination that so many people face. Central to *Time to Change* is that more and more people are now speaking out and telling their own stories so that more people can find out more about mental health both as a condition and how we can help – and sometimes hinder – individuals' recovery.

In the summer of 2009, Professor Steve Boorman published the review of the health and well-being of the NHS workforce. In his interim report, he has highlighted the need to improve the mental health support of staff who develop mental health conditions. There is sometimes an additional fear, and an additional stigma amongst health staff, to find and access health services for themselves, so this recognition by the NHS is important.

For all these reasons, the timing of Veronica Burton's book, chronicling her own experiences, could not be more important. As someone with direct experience of depression, she is able to explain in great detail the journey that millions of people go on, and the impact it had on her and her friends. As an employee of the NHS, she has highlighted the additional stresses that she faced.

I hope that many people will read this book, both within and outside the NHS, so that we can continue to tackle stigma and discrimination, and fight for the right for people who experience mental health problems to be treated as equal citizens in our society.

Paul Farmer
Chief Executive, Mind
November 2009

Preface

This book centres on my experience of major depression, many hospital admissions and treatments including medication, electro-convulsive therapy (ECT) and 'talking treatments'. My first experience came when I was a teenager. I had a ten-year remission during which time I was able to gain my general nursing qualification. I worked at the neonatal unit in High Wycombe and I completed my Special and Intensive Nursing of the Newborn course at the John Radcliffe Hospital in Oxford. I became a confident practitioner with real faith in my abilities at work. In 1988 a system was introduced to pay nurses according to grades as allocated. I appealed against the grading I received. No doubt I was rather naive then; I ignored warnings from the unit senior sister that appealing would make me rather unpopular. I went ahead and as a result the weight of the hospital management came down on me. At the grading appeal, and afterwards, I saw the spectacle of my supposed superiors fabricate evidence, tell blatant lies and lose evidence in the form of personnel records (twice, apparently – very careless). The treatment that I received at work was directly responsible for my depressive relapse, which has so far lasted nineteen years.

I discuss the care given to me by medical and nursing staff – the fact that I was a nurse made it very difficult to cope with being cared for by psychiatric colleagues. It was something that I was very sensitive about, especially during my initial admissions to hospital.

My experience of psychiatric illness made me very aware of prejudice. I combined with another nurse, Ian Payne, to stage a two-nurse campaign against prejudice towards nurses (including mental health nurses) who need psychological support of any kind, by their own colleagues. I fear there is still work to be done on this matter.

I relate the success, or otherwise, of treatments including medication and ECT.

My main source for information has been my journal, kept through all that time. I have some extracts from my health records. I have a file with all papers relevant to the events in High Wycombe following the grading exercise, from which I have quoted in the text.

Veronica Burton
November 2009

About the author

As a teenager I suffered serious depression. I recovered and went to Durham University, graduating in 1982. I then qualified as a nurse. I descended into deep depression in 1989. I had many admissions to a psychiatric hospital while the depression remained persistent. Despite this, I managed to gain my paediatric nursing and other qualifications. However, I was medically retired from nursing in 1995.

As a nurse I discovered the depth of prejudice against mental illness among nursing and medical personnel. A fellow nurse and I fought to show the extent of this problem. We highlighted something that was previously taboo.

I have lived in the Oxford area for many years, but am moving to Salisbury, my family home for generations.

Acknowledgements

I am particularly grateful to Gillian Nineham at Radcliffe Publishing, for her invaluable help and guidance, and to Ollie Judkin and Jamie Etherington. Thanks also to Camille Lowe of Pindar NZ.

Many thanks to Jack Salter and Wendy Benson for preparing and processing the photographs that have been included. To my other friends from prayer breakfast, and those in my church house group, for their encouragement and interest.

My sister Jane, also a writer, has been a helpful source of advice and guidance. Throughout all the years I have suffered this illness, Diana has always been there. My thanks to my mother for her understanding, having had depression herself. I am greatly saddened that my father died before he could see this book.

I am deeply grateful for the care I have received from psychiatric nursing and medical staff, and my GP, Dr Price. I also appreciate the support given to me by the various occupational health (OH) departments which I attended, particularly the OH consultant and senior nurse at High Wycombe. Other professionals involved include physiotherapists, occupational therapists, housekeepers, Anne and Elaine, the hairdressers, and many others – they all had their role. Dr Nicholas Rose, psychiatric consultant, and Tim Woodward, mental health nurse, for encouraging me to write for publication. And to all those whom I cannot fully acknowledge in these few words.

I have changed many, but not all names. Nurses are referred to by their names where I have been able to obtain their permission, or given pseudonyms. A notable exception is that of Tim Ackland, who was tragically killed in an accident, a great loss, not least to mental health nursing. I hope that what I have written about him is some form of tribute.

My friends and relatives are given their real names in all instances.

To the memory of Kathleen Cooper (1994–2007).
A greatly supportive friend who always believed in me.

Written in Northamptonshire County Asylum

I AM! yet what I am who cares, or knows?
My friends forsake me like a memory lost.
I am the self-consumer of my woes;
They rise and vanish, an oblivious host,
Shadows of life, whose very soul is lost.
And yet I am – I lie – though I am tossed

Into the nothingness of scorn and noise,
Into the living sea of waking dream,
Where there is neither sense of life, nor joys,
But the huge shipwreck of my own esteem
And all that's dear. Even those I loved the best
Are strange – nay, they are stranger than the rest.

I long for scenes where man has never trod –
For scenes where never woman smiled nor wept –
There to abide with my Creator, God;
And sleep as I in childhood sweetly slept
Full of high thoughts, unborn. So let me lie, –
The grass below; above, the vaulted sky.

John Clare (1793–1864)

Chapter 1

Childhood in Salisbury – School

'Oh, come on, and stop complaining,' Peter told Patrick. Having to take his younger brother and sisters out was not his idea of fun at the best of times; he could do without all this fuss. They were never going to get home.

We had been catching minnows from the river, about two miles from home. Not long after we had started for home, we had had to climb over a stile. Patrick had jumped off the stile and given a shriek of pain as he landed.

'I can't walk!' Patrick declared.

'Well, how do you think we are to get home if you don't walk?' Peter said, rather unsympathetically. Despite Peter's exhortations, progress was slow but eventually we arrived. Mother asked Patrick how he had hurt his leg. Pat explained about his jump from the stile. Mother looked at it and immediately decided that he would have to go to casualty. She took him to catch the bus.

When Patrick returned, some considerable time later, he had a half-leg plaster and two crutches. We were impressed. He even said that we could write on the plaster. 'The doctor didn't know what a stile was,' he told us, with considerable amusement. '"Stile? What is this stile?" he asked.' The idea that someone did not know what a stile was met with general laughter.

My brother Patrick was very clever; he could say the whole alphabet and do up his own shoelaces. He was already big enough to snatch a straw from the thatched wall in the village of Stratford-sub-Castle. The castle in question was Old Sarum, which overlooked the village. We liked to kick the thatched wall because there were pig sties the other side and it made the pigs squeal. The path alongside the farm and down to the river was called 'stink pot alley' by us, as it had been by my father and his friends as children. The pig farm is no longer and the site of the pig sties now has large houses on it.

Old Sarum has impressive ancient earthworks around it, having a moat around the central castle and another around the site itself; we called them 'the rings'. We would take sledges to the outer moat and career down the steep slope trying, sometimes unsuccessfully, to avoid being pitched into one of the small but painful thorn bushes on the slope. Sometimes, on a hot summer's day, Mother would come with us and sit on a rug doing her knitting while we played our usual games. One of our favourite areas of the outer moat was where it was covered in immense beech trees. Sometimes we were able to take advantage of a rope to swing on, one that older children had tied to a tree branch. The moat was high and steep at this point but we could get up it by using the protruding roots as hand and foot holds. One of my young nephews tried it recently but, on looking down, got scared and would go no further. I went to rescue him, telling him what to hold onto and where to put his feet, so he managed to get to the top. At his age, we would have scrambled up without a thought.

There were the medieval remains of the cathedral crypt. We used to scramble over the walls and climb down into it. This was before English Heritage took over the site and there were proper wooden steps to the bottom, and signs forbidding climbing on the walls.

We would spend hours wandering the fields and villages around, always finding something to entertain us. Having generally been told not to come home until teatime, we stayed out all afternoon whatever the weather. We had a wonderful degree of freedom. None of us having watches, we would approach a likely adult and politely ask if they had the time. 'There's no excuse for bad manners,' my mother frequently told us.

It was not, of course, all idyllic. When we were little, we would often come home crying because we were cold and the older ones had walked us too far. Conversely, our older brother and sisters would often complain that they could go nowhere without a younger sibling or two in tow.

It was not too long before all our elder brothers and sisters left home. Jane went to university in Durham, a considerable achievement; no one else in our family had ever been to university, and certainly not to Durham. When my father had gained a place at the grammar school in Salisbury, his father would not let him take it up. He believed that you left school and got a proper job, so my father had to leave at fourteen to work in a cobbler's. I wonder what would have happened if he had taken the place up, as he was essentially a very intelligent man, but his abilities had never been tested. When he was in the Post Office, he came second out of the entire West Country in an examination for post office clerks. He did the job for a while, then left and returned to being a postman as he simply could not cope with the responsibility of being behind the counter. He certainly had the ability, but his upbringing had done nothing to imbue him with any confidence.

Fortunately, my parents did not take the view my grandfather had; education was important to them, particularly to my mother. One thing we had in our house, that none of the children in the council houses around us had, was books. Our house was full of books. We all learned to read early and were voracious readers. My father would buy books for us from Beeches, the second-hand bookshop, and whenever he was home at our bedtime, he would read us a story. I can remember him reading *Children of the New Forest* and the Narnia books to us.

Mother was quite formidable when she took on a campaign, such as persuading the County Council that they should pay for Catholic children to go to La Retraite Convent, the private Roman Catholic school. My father always said that you could introduce Mother to the Queen and she would just start chatting. Her attitude was very much that she was as good as anyone else, and that was what she passed onto us. At the hospital, where she worked as a nursing auxiliary, she was on friendly terms with everyone from the cleaners to senior management and consultants.

My father used to tell us that if we had a question to go ahead and ask it, even if our classmates laughed – those that laughed were often the ones who wanted to know the answer. We were encouraged to stand up for ourselves and have the courage of our convictions.

Something else that distinguished us from the children who lived around us was the fact that we were always clean and well dressed. Both our parents were always well turned out. We used to complain about Mother's insisting that we wore our good clothes whenever we went into town. She would always tell us, 'You might meet someone I know.' That was certainly a likelihood, as Mother has always seemed to know half the city or more. She got to know so many people because, basically, she was interested in people and always enjoyed talking to them.

Diana went to Southampton to work in a children's home, then came back to Salisbury to start her nurse training. I can remember her bringing one of the little boys she looked after in Southampton, to Salisbury, for a trip out. Diana's departure left us younger four – Patrick, me, Clare and Eleanor – at home without the elder four. I then had to take on the domestic chores, as my parents were both working. Patrick was the eldest but Mother always said, 'Girls are more sensible than boys.'

Clare was eighteen months younger than me. She and I were always great rivals as children and Clare usually insisted on being uncooperative and making things difficult for me. On the whole, however, Patrick supported me. One day though, he decided to join Clare and I became so angry and frustrated that I told them they could cook their own meal. I got on my bike and cycled for about twenty miles. Eventually I stopped by the side of the road and thought about the situation. I became suddenly scared that the others might have some accident and set the house alight. They might all die and it would be my fault. I turned around and cycled home even more quickly than I had cycled away. Needless to say, they were fine. Patrick just told me that my dinner was in the oven. I, however, was always plagued by an oppressive sense of responsibility.

Sometimes Father was at home at a weekend and cooked for us. His specialty on a Saturday was bangers and mash. He would sing at the full strength of his powerful voice, *give us a bash at the bangers and mash my mama used to make!*, whereupon we would shout in unison 'Daddy! Shut up!' and he would always laugh. He could also make a decent roast dinner if he was at home on a Sunday. He was unusual as a man of that time as he would happily take on domestic chores, like the vacuum cleaning and the ironing. I was always quite close to my father, as my mother once said to me, 'you always had a special relationship with him'.

On graduating, Jane married John and they lived in Essex. Jane taught English. My brother Jon had left home but would come back at Christmas and put up the decorations and the Christmas tree for us. Peter went into the army, the Parachute Regiment, going successfully through the famously challenging training despite those who foretold that he would never stick it. Diana married Pete Cameron and they lived initially in a flat in Castle Street, where they would have Clare and me to stay. We were at junior school at the time. We could have toast at Diana's, as she had the luxury of a toaster; the only time we could have it at home was in the winter and there was a fire for us to toast the bread on, but there is something special about fire-toasted bread. In term time, Diana would give us a chocolate biscuit for a snack at break time, which was a real treat.

Whenever there was a craze at school – I remember that once it was for packs of fifty coloured felt pens – we had to resign ourselves to not joining in. We accepted that our parents could not afford such things and did not ask for them. One day, when I was at my senior school, La Retraite Convent, a school trip to Greece was announced to see the ancient sites. I would have loved to have gone, for I really enjoyed my classics lessons, but I dismissed the idea immediately and did not mention it to my parents. However, Sister Mary, the classics teacher, saw Mother at a parents' evening and told her that of all the pupils in the school I would gain the most from going. At home, my father explained that he thought he could pay subsequent instalments but the trouble was producing the initial £20 deposit at short notice. However, he contacted my brother Peter, who sent him the money by return of post. Each of my elder brothers and sisters gave me spending money.

I had loved classics ever since I had first read Roger Lancelyn-Greene's *Tales of the Greek Heroes*. By the time I went to La Retraite, I had an impressive knowledge of the classical civilisations, particularly Greek. Sister Mary, recognising that I already knew what she was teaching, used to recommend books to me and allow me to read them at the back, while she taught the rest of the class. One day she had to leave the classroom to take a telephone call and left the room saying that I could finish off the story for them. At first I was uncertain – did my classmates really want to learn the Greek myths from me? However, they urged me to continue and so I did, completing the story by the time Sister Mary returned.

At Durham, Dr Black, who taught Greek mythology on the classics course I did, soon found out the extent of my knowledge and thereafter used to tell me to be quiet whenever I opened my mouth to answer a question. 'Be quiet,' he would say, 'you know too much' and 'No – let them answer it'.

One of the classics lecturers told us not to ask him questions – he got all his information from Dr Black on coffee breaks. Rather sadly I think, I've forgotten most of what I knew then, but it was thirty years ago. In the end, I was able to go on the school trip and was enchanted by all I saw.

Maureen Macdonald was a teacher who had a lasting effect on me. I am still in touch with my old school friend Sue. She commented to me, not so long ago, that it was Mrs Macdonald who had the greatest influence on her becoming a Christian. Mrs Macdonald had a similar effect on me. She was our religious studies teacher and was very clear about moral standards on, for instance, racism. It was made quite plain to us that we should never judge anyone by the colour of their skin. She not only taught us Christian values, she lived by them herself.

One thing that we hated at home was the rows between our parents. I suspect it was all that shouting that made me so very sensitive to noise and hateful of the sound of slamming doors or raised voices. It was tragic that my parents were so unhappy together.

I went to stay with Diana quite often. Even before she and Pete were married, I would often be tagging along with them. I always think that Pete was remarkably tolerant, having his girlfriend's little sister with them so often. About three days a week, I would go to Di's straight after school. She and Pete moved to a little terraced house on the outskirts of the city centre. Pete then got a house through his work, just up the hill from the family home in Castle Road. When it was decided to sell the houses, Pete and Diana were able to buy their house.

Patrick, Clare and I went to St Martin's Church of England School, while Eleanor, for some reason, was sent to St Osmund's Catholic School. Our headmaster at St Martin's was Mr Allen. He would play the piano while we sang. Occasionally he would stop playing, then, when we dried up, would admonish us for stopping singing. One day I decided that I would not be fooled and so, when he stopped playing, I went on singing to the end of the song, all on my own. Mr Allen sat back and listened. When I came to the end he said, 'That was lovely! Who was it?'

I was horrified. I had only intended to show that he could not catch me out. He asked again and the boy next to me – I can still remember his name – started trying to encourage me to own up, even taking my hand to try to raise it. I dare not say anything in case I were to attract attention to myself, but I gesticulated frantically at him to stop making a fuss. Mr Allen never did discover who the singer was.

I had started at my senior school, La Retraite Convent, in 1971. We were able to go to the Convent, paid for by the County, because of Mother's campaign to allow children from Catholic families to have their fees paid if they passed the 11+ exam. I surprised everyone by passing; for some reason, it had been thought I would fail. Jane and Diana had been to La Retraite before me, so my family was well known. They had both left, however, by the time I arrived. One year, there were three of us at La Retraite together – Clare, Eleanor and me. Eleanor was in the first year while I was in the sixth form.

When I first went to La Retraite (or 'Colditz', as Clare called it) I had a problem that puzzled me. I was continually being asked to repeat myself. What was wrong? Were they deaf, or something? Gradually, the truth dawned on me – they could not understand my Wiltshire dialect. I carefully cultivated the Queen's English, or 'received pronunciation' as it is called. To this day, however, there are words I still pronounce in a good Moonraker fashion. Just recently, my GP asked me when my community nurse was next going to visit. 'T'marrr'o,' I replied.

She looked puzzled, so I repeated what I had said. 'You mean he's not coming?' she asked hesitantly.

I realised what the problem was. It was Tuesday, so I said, 'Wednesday. Sorry, I come from Wiltshire.'

The Convent was a small school. There were two classes in each year, but we often did things together, such as swimming, for which we had to be particularly hardy as at that time the only pool was an outdoor one – less than inviting on a wet or overcast day. There was another Veronica in the other class of my year. It was actually the first time that I had come across anyone with that good Catholic name, no doubt because I had gone to a Church of England junior school.

I remember one girl in particular, who joined us in the fifth form. Her father was a company director. One day she asked me what my father did and I told her that he was a postman. Apparently she went and asked one of my friends if this was true – she could not believe that the daughter of a postman could be top of the class at the end of almost every term. Postmen's daughters were not clever.

We had a very patriotic Scotswoman for a geography teacher. One day she made some caustic comment about Prince Charles hiding in an oak tree and said that in Scotland, they did not go hiding like that. 'No,' I said in response, 'I understand you skulk in caves up there.' She was actually persuaded to smile.

I could walk across the downs from the Convent to Diana and Pete's, which I did regularly three times a week. By this time they had baby Jim and I would often baby-sit while they went out for a drink, usually with Pete's friend Pete Day, who had known Pete from school days, and was a frequent visitor.

The headmistress who was at La Retraite when Clare and I were first there was someone who commanded great respect. She was incredibly understanding; an attribute demonstrated to me when I was in the second form. She met me in an empty corridor, stopped me, and asked if there was anything wrong. I shook my head, denying it. She accepted this, though I suspected that she was not satisfied. One day, not long after, she entered our classroom and we all rose to our feet. To my confusion, she had come in to ask me to go to her office with her. She sat behind her desk, inviting me to sit opposite.

She then explained that the teachers were worried about me as I seemed very unhappy. This was unusual, as I was usually the form joker and kept the teachers and my fellow pupils laughing. The headmistress asked me what was wrong. I burst into tears and said, 'My brother's in Ireland.' Soldiers seemed to be getting killed almost daily at that time, in the 1970s. I was desperately worried about Peter and had had nightmares for the first time since I was a child. I wrote a letter every week – which is a good deal more than you can say of Peter!

It was that same headmistress who took me into her office to tell me that my parents were about to go through a divorce. She said that I would find it hard as I was an idealist. In the event they separated but did not divorce.

I was successful in my 'O' levels. I took the first, English language, in 1975, and the rest in the long, hot summer of 1976. With my two closest friends, Sue and Carol, I went camping on my uncle's farm in Cornwall. When I returned to school in the sixth form it was without Sue or Carol, who had always been with me at La Retraite, as their families had moved away. Although the great majority of the girls who went into the sixth form with me had followed me through from the first year, and we all got on well, I still felt bereft without my special friends.

My mother had gone through a period of major depression, which gave her an appreciation of how depression could affect you. She remained understanding throughout my illness. However, my parents' separation caused me great distress. In addition, during my teenage years – when establishing your own identity is so important – this was difficult for me being a member of such a close, large family. As an adult I greatly value my family, but I first had to find myself as an individual, to value my separateness. These things all had their effect.

Chapter 2

Meningitis – Depression – Help from brother-in-law's friend
and GP – 'A' levels

In August 1976, I was sixteen and due to start my two-year 'A' levels
course. I returned after the summer holidays to the absence of my
closest friends from school. I think this was part of the reason why
I became steadily depressed, though I did not recognise what was
happening; I was just aware of being supremely miserable. I continued to go to Diana's several times a week, as I always had. One
day my brother-in-law's friend, Pete Day, a psychiatric nurse, and I
were alone in the sitting room. Pete took the opportunity to say to
me, 'If you want someone to talk to, you know where I am.'

It was not until he said that that I realised how desperately I
needed to talk to someone as sympathetic and understanding as
Pete proved to be. I amazed myself at how extreme and negative
my thoughts were – nothing was any good, there was no point in
trying to help me, nothing would ever improve anything, I could
not do anything right, it was all disastrous, it would not matter if
I was not there anymore as no one would miss me – negativity and
catastrophising, two major aspects of depressive thought. I began to
live for those days when I could leave school and cycle over to Pete's

flat and could talk about things that surprised even me. Pete tried to persuade me to see my GP, but I consistently refused on the grounds that he would only give me tablets and I would not take any.

One day I became very distressed and started to hyperventilate. Pete sat back and waited for the fit to end. When I had calmed down, he told me that I was really too ill for him to cope with alone and I must go to see my GP. As before, he told me that Dr Hamber was also his doctor and he was sure that he would be sympathetic.

I made an appointment to see Dr Hamber, but told no one except Pete. When I entered his surgery, he had a student with him. I asked him if I could see him alone, to which he readily agreed. The student went out and I was left to explain myself. I told him how Pete had helped me and how he had advised me to go to see him. Dr Hamber asked me about my sleep, my thoughts and other such things. When he had finished questioning me, he explained that he thought I was too unwell for him to manage so he would send me to see a specialist. He said that he would refer me to the Child Guidance Clinic, rather than the adult services which he did not feel would be appropriate. I was only just sixteen anyway. I found Dr Hamber wonderfully sympathetic.

When I was next at Diana's, I realised that she had found out that I had been seeing Pete and was upset that I had not told her. I dissolved into tears, feeling terrible that I'd upset her, but seeing how upset I was, she forgave me. She came with me to see the psychiatrist at the Clinic. I can remember little of what happened at that meeting, except that the psychiatrist said I would have to leave the family home. Too many people and too much happening. At the time my father was staying with Di and Pete, as my parents were going through a separation. He agreed to move out for me to live with Di. I was lucky; I don't know what would have happened if Father had not recognised that my needs were greater or what they would have done with me if I had not been able to live with Di and Pete.

I continued to see Pete Day, and saw Dr Hamber on a weekly basis. I can remember little about visits to the psychiatrist. I remember one day going to school and feeling awful. I asked to see Mrs Macdonald and she took me to the 'chicken parlour'. I was in an extremely distressed state. Mrs Mac asked me to stay where I was then left me for a while. She came back with Sr Mary, who was then the headmistress. She took me to the Bishop's Room where there was a bed I was able to lay on. One of the nuns came and sat with me and did not leave until another came to relieve her. I was not left alone all day. Eventually Sr Mary returned and took me in the convent's car to the Clinic, where I saw the psychiatrist. I realised that Sr Mary must have been following his instructions in ensuring that I was not left alone. I had admitted to feeling suicidal and they were obviously not taking any chances.

The psychiatrist wanted to admit me to hospital but Dr Hamber would not agree to that unless they could find a place in an adolescent unit. He felt that the Old Manor, with its highly disturbed patients and locked wards, was not the place for a teenager. Apparently Oxford was the nearest place with an adolescent unit, but they did not have any beds. Neither had any of the other places that Dr Hamber tried.

The situation became further complicated as I became obsessed with my weight and what I ate. I would record, several times a day, what I had eaten including, literally, every little crumb I had consumed and estimated the calories represented – a crumb counted as one calorie, but was nevertheless included – and I invariably got worried that I had eaten too much. Despite my obsessive avoidance of eating, I became fanatical about feeding others. I was often cooking; food which I would never eat myself. I would weigh myself every day and only be satisfied if my weight had gone down. Dr Hamber would get me to stand on the scales when he saw me each week, give a slight sigh, and record the ever-decreasing weight. One day I asked him what was wrong and he explained anorexia nervosa to me. At that time, in the 1970s, anorexia nervosa was not the well-known illness that it is today, nor as common. I had not heard of it before. I do not know why I was so affected by it, as I had always been very slim and had never tried to lose weight before. My depression was such that I never read the magazines that featured diets and ultra-thin models.

One morning in February 1977, I got up for school with a headache. I insisted that I was all right to go to school. The headache was getting quickly and progressively worse. I decided not to go to morning assembly. The first lesson was double English. I explained to the teacher that I had a bad headache and I simply sat with my head in my arms on the desk for the entire lesson. The teacher came up to me at the end of class and asked me if I was all right and I assured her I was. She did not seem entirely convinced. By the end of the first break time, my headache had got sufficiently worse for even me to admit it was becoming near unbearable. I met one of the teachers outside the staff room and asked her if she could get Mrs Macdonald, my sixth form tutor, whom I had asked for as my tutor myself. She knew my family well and had always been highly complimentary about me and I had always found her an excellent teacher.

While I was waiting for her, I literally sat on a radiator as I had started to feel cold and shivery. One of my classmates came down the corridor, looked at me and said, 'Veronica, you're white! Are you all right?' I assured her, no doubt rather unconvincingly, that I was.

Mrs Macdonald came and I told her I was feeling ill and thought I ought to go home. She offered to drive me, but I said I would be fine and insisted on walking the mile home. Once I got there, I did not go to bed but sat in a chair. It was one of the days that I went to my sister Diana's after school (before I went to live there) and I did not intend to miss that. Father came in for dinner (midday meal, we were not posh enough for lunch in those days). He was obviously concerned when he saw me, and things were by then bad enough for me to be persuaded to go to bed.

As the afternoon went on, I became unwell enough to have to admit that I needed a doctor. Mother had come home and tried to reassure me, yet when she looked at the thermometer she had just taken out of my mouth she did not tell me the reading but called for Patrick to go to the telephone box and phone the doctor. She then decided that she had better go herself. The situation was obviously serious.

My own GP was not available but one of the others in the practice came. Mother has never forgiven him for not making a diagnosis that evening. He was, however, sufficiently concerned to return the next morning. He then told my mother that he suspected meningitis and would call an ambulance to admit me to hospital. I was very ill by then and the pain had progressed down my spine. Both times the doctor came, he took my head in his hands and bent my neck to take my chin towards my chest. He then bent my leg at the knee and the hip then straightened it out. This elicited a positive Kernig's sign – in other words, it was very painful. I was confused and wondered why he was inflicting this pain on me. They did the same thing in casualty, then kept repeating it when I was on the ward. I could not understand why they insisted on causing that pain. My thought processes were not by then sufficient for me to come to the conclusion that they were monitoring the development of the illness. Before they sent me to the ward, they sat me up for an X-ray, whereupon I promptly vomited. Served them right for sitting me up.

I had to have a lumbar puncture, in which cerebro-spinal fluid was taken from my spine with a large needle. Fortunately the doctor who did it gave the local anaesthetic enough time to work before she proceeded. The sample was sent away and, once the diagnosis was verified, I was transferred from the infirmary in town to the isolation unit at Odstock Hospital, some three miles out in the country. I was told it would be quiet for me there – so they put me in the room opposite the sluice and bedpan washer, and the telephone extension. It was before the hospice movement had demonstrated that it was possible to give adequate pain relief without getting the patient addicted. I was given two distaelgesic for the journey, which was utterly inadequate. Every bump we went over sent a searing pain along my spine to my head.

One thing amazed me – I desperately wanted my mother. After all, I was a teenager, I was self-sufficient, or so I thought. When they transferred me, I was really worried that my mother would not know where I was. The simple fact that the ward staff would tell her did not occur to my bewildered mind. I was very relieved when the ambulance men took me on to Sarum Ward at Odstock. She was having a cup of tea with the nurses, whom she knew well as she had worked on that ward. Over the following days she would come to visit me and wipe my face and hands with a cool flannel, which I found quite comforting.

I had been admitted on the Friday and moved to Odstock on the Saturday. Jane, my eldest sister, telephoned my brother Peter's home barracks where, fortunately, he was then stationed. Unsurprisingly Peter was out with his mates on a Saturday evening, so Jane left a message at the guardhouse.

Sunday morning the night nurse came into my room about seven o'clock, as usual. 'Your brother's here,' she told me.

'Which one?' I asked, though I knew it could only be Peter.

'The one who's in the army,' the nurse replied. 'He's been here since four o'clock.'

They allowed Peter to come in to see me for a short while. He sat by my bed, and almost apologetically told me that he had got Jane's message after the final train had gone, so he decided to hitchhike. It was a freezing February night and he had not even gone home first but had come directly to the hospital.

The next morning a large, beautiful bouquet was brought in by one of the nurses. 'Who's it from?' I asked.

'That's funny,' the nurse said, 'there's no name on the card.'

'Oh, that will be Peter.'

After I came out of hospital, Mrs Macdonald had me to stay so that I could have some peace and quiet. She and her husband were both very kind to me and looked after me well. I was still having quite severe headaches.

My depression meant that I was not exposed to the normal teenage experiences. I never had boyfriends or knew what it was like to have a break-up of such a relationship. If I ever went to a disco, I would usually wander outside and sit on my own. I never joined in with the others and to this day nothing will induce me to take part in a disco or go onto the disco dance floor. I never wore make-up, so what I know of making up your face came from what I learned from my fellow students at Durham. Even now I rarely wear it, though that is not entirely owing to the shortcomings of my teenage years. I'm not the sort of person to wear make-up all the time, though I certainly went up to Durham not knowing anything about how to use it.

I began to exercise manically, even running on the spot in my room rather than standing still. I would cycle sometimes forty miles a day and would run rather than walk. How I got the energy I will never know, for I was eating next to nothing. I became gradually more devious about avoiding food and convincing Diana or my mother that I was eating, how successfully I do not know. Since I was ill I have never discussed it, though one day Diana asked me if I realised that she put Build-Up in my drinking chocolate at night. I did not. I wondered, did she realise that most of it went down the sink?

I felt ashamed of the scheming and devious measures I took to avoid food and I am sure that that is one of the main reasons I have never been able to discuss it. It started in autumn 1976 and by the time I started at university in 1979 I was eating more, but I continued to choose salads and to be afraid of eating too much. I became literally afraid of having to eat and worried desperately when I gave in to the need for food.

Complete recovery came slowly and took a long time.

The causes of anorexia nervosa are usually given as the obsession in the media with ultra-thin models and the popularity of dieting and diets. But I had never tried a diet in my life. Another theory sees it as an attempt to avoid growing up and maturing. I think that had more relevance for me. Ironically, perhaps, I had too much responsibility too early and was afraid of attracting more.

Through all this time I was very depressed. I was prescribed a hypnotic by the psychiatrist to help me sleep, but it had little effect. I would spend the nights sitting up, lying down, rolling on to one side then the other, not knowing what to do with myself. I was plagued by the most appallingly dark and suicidal thoughts. I had a strange and disturbing feeling, as if I had a large ball stuck in my gullet. I kept swallowing to try to get rid of the feeling but nothing would take the horrible experience away.

I continued to go to school and worked as if possessed. I did not get very good 'A' level results, despite this. Durham accepted me as a result of a letter pleading my case from Sr Mary, herself a Durham graduate, and on the strength of my 'O' level results.

Physically my illness was having an effect. My hair began to fall out, as my mother observed one day. I was amenorrhoeic and my extreme thinness resulted in my being constantly cold, so the many layers I wore were not simply to hide my emaciation. In the spring of 1977 I developed pneumonia and was off school again. My mother commented that she was surprised it had not carried me off.

Those teenage years were, I decided, the worst in all my life.

Chapter 3

University – I meet Richard – Depressed patient while I am on night duty – SCBU grading and appeal – Richard's mother comes to stay – I see Hugh Wilson, rector of High Wycombe, to talk to him about the way I am feeling – Suicidal/depressed thoughts – I telephone Hugh, who telephones the doctor

When I initially applied to Durham, they suggested that I take a year out, as I was still not entirely fit. Anyway, as they pointed out, I was young to start a university course, seventeen when I applied. I therefore went away and worked for a year, initially as a nanny/mother's help caring for three children, then returned to Salisbury as a nursing auxiliary. I then went up to Durham in 1979.

Richard was in the third year of a maths course at Durham when I was in my first year. He had a great sense of humour and could always make me laugh. He was also very generous, something my mother remembers him for even now. He was very affectionate towards me.

He and I shared a love of classical music. At home, I would often listen to Radio Three when I was alone in the dining room. With Richard, I experienced the delight of going to classical concerts. One year my sister and brother-in-law were away during some of the Proms weeks and said that we could stay in their house at Purley so that we could go into London to attend the Proms. Richard took a lot of persuading that it was all right to stay in someone's house while they were away. He had no experience of sisters or brothers, so my explanation that Jane was my sister and trusted me to look after her house meant nothing to him. In the end he agreed to come, however. Richard always paid for the tickets and got some of the best – and most expensive – seats. This was new to my experience.

I met Richard's parents when they came to Durham and took us out to lunch. I got on with them very well. I was somewhat amazed, however, the first time I went to his house. All four of us were seated watching television, when Richard looked at his mother and said, 'Mum, can I have a coffee?' That he should ask his mother and not get up to get his own drink surprised me enough, but what followed was even more astounding. She actually stopped watching the television, went to the kitchen and made the coffee as requested. My mother would have said, 'Yes – and I'll have one too.'

I was going for a short walk with Richard one day, when he said that he could never spend Christmas away from his parents. I was astonished – would his parents really demand his presence every Christmas, even if he were married? I was slowly getting the picture of his relationship with his parents. Annie, his mother, spoke as if she had given him everything, asking nothing in return. However, she brought to my mind a quote said to be from Alexander the Great, who apparently commented of his mother, 'She demands a high rent for nine months' lodging.' Annie certainly demanded a great deal from Richard. More, I think, than his father, she demanded everything of him. This became evident after his father's death – she would demand his full attention. I soon came to recognise a particular expression she used whenever she threatened to get upset if Richard did not behave precisely as she wished him to. Richard seemed to be equally afraid of upsetting his mother.

As I became increasingly aware of the hold Annie had over him and considering Richard's statements, such as that he would have to spend every Christmas with his parents, I became quite concerned. Did I really want to take on Richard's parents along with him? I was highly dubious about that but the more I thought of it, the more I became worried that if I left Richard no one else would ever care for me. All my own insecurities came out when I considered returning to life on my own, and I became very anxious. I was consciously afraid of being alone for the rest of my life. Anyway, I loved him.

I went to Durham for Congregation (graduation, Durham likes to be different), when Richard received his degree. I was unable to go into the ceremony as Richard was given only three tickets – for his parents and for him. Before my Congregation, I got in touch with administration and got two extra tickets, free of charge, one for my sister Jane, who drove my mother and father to Durham, and one for Richard. I could have seen Richard receive his degree if he had done likewise, but he did not. I do not know why. It was probably a simple lack of initiative.

On graduating, Richard took up a job in the Midlands and went to live in that area. I joined him in the holidays, though he refused to tell his parents of the situation, something that I was unhappy about. When I left Durham, I joined him and we supposedly became engaged – in retrospect I can appreciate that this, Richard's suggestion, was really a way of keeping me with him at a time when I was considering doing post-graduate courses elsewhere. Given that he consistently refused to give me any date for actually getting married, I can only assume that keeping me with him was the most important aspect. While we were still in the Midlands, I started nurse training – something to which Richard was opposed, but it had always been a possibility in my mind. I transferred to High Wycombe halfway through my training, as Richard took a new job there.

Before we moved, I was working nights and came across a patient I have never forgotten. My friend Kathy and I were on the same ward, a male medical ward. This particular night there was a patient who had been transferred from the intensive care unit. He had quite fortuitously been found in some woods, having taken a noxious cocktail of medication and cleaning chemicals. There can hardly have been any doubt that he meant to kill himself, but they had resuscitated him and taken him to intensive care. He was due to go to the psychiatric hospital the morning after his night on the medical ward.

I watched him and have never seen anyone betraying such extreme distress. He did not know what to do with himself; he would sit up, lie down, turn on one side, then the other, sit up again with his legs drawn up and his face in his hands. I could sit and watch him any longer. I went over to him, took his hand in mine, and talked to him. He clutched at my hand with tears running down his face, telling me that no one had ever talked to him like I did. He said that he could not understand how someone so young could be so understanding. I did not tell him. There are times when it is wrong to burden a patient with your own experiences.

I went back to the desk and was relieved to see that he lay down and actually went to sleep. Kathy said, 'You were fantastic, I would have hit him over the head.' I doubt if she was the only one who had felt like hitting him over the head, after all, nurses, doctors and NHS facilities were there for those who were genuinely ill, not attention-seekers like that man. I felt angry. What right had they to drag him back from the dead, then congratulate themselves and blame him? Kathy later surprised herself by enjoying her psychiatric second-ment. She was very supportive of me throughout my depression. Once I moved away, we would have long telephone conversations and I always found what Kathy said to be very encouraging.

It was just before we left the area that Richard's father died. I was very upset by this, as he had always been kind to me, but Richard in his grief failed to notice the affect it had on me. He was very distressed.

His mother had stopped work as soon as she married, a skilled job painting gold onto pottery in Stoke-on-Trent. After her mar-riage, she did not do anything like joining in local activities, doing voluntary work or joining an organisation such as the Women's Institute; she simply did the housework and waited for her husband to come home. They were living in a north country village when Richard was at Durham. She once told me that she used to go into the nearby town simply to talk to the shop girls.

She had Richard late in life (long before in-vitro fertilisation – IVF), having had to undergo pioneering surgery. Richard was the miracle baby and Annie was ridiculously protective of him as he grew up. He was not even allowed to lose at snakes and ladders. When his father died, Richard was all his mother had. Although I had got on well with her before her husband died, I was soon to dis-cover that she could be very manipulative, especially when it came to getting Richard's attention.

We lived in a rented flat in High Wycombe as we waited for the flat in the Midlands to sell. Richard actually admitted to his mother that we were living together and invited her to stay with us for two weeks. I had no objections to this – I was yet to discover what a trial her presence could be.

I particularly remember the day I was to be confirmed into the Anglican Church. This was very important to me; I had come to be very dissatisfied with the Catholic Church and found that I dis-agreed with too much of Catholic doctrine to be comfortable in that Church. My faith was too important for me to be content with compromising. I had therefore gone to Hugh Wilson, rector of High Wycombe and vicar of All Saints, the church in High Wycombe that I attended. My sister Jane and brother-in-law John, and my mother, had come to attend the service. I was going to read one of the lessons but had not told Richard, as I wanted to give him a surprise. In the event it was I who had the surprise. Just before we were going, Annie, who was supposed to be coming too, said that she was not feeling well. Richard decided he would have to stay with her and so was not present at what was, for me, a very important ceremony. When we got back, Annie was quite all right despite her supposed illness. This was just the start of what I found to be a very strong hold that she had over Richard and which she was never adverse to exerting.

Her two-week stay had presented so many difficulties for me that when Richard suggested she stay with us indefinitely (by now the flat in the Midlands had been sold, enabling us to buy a house in Chinnor, between High Wycombe and Oxford) while she found somewhere to live near us; I immediately protested. In the end I gave in, however, and Annie came to stay.

I qualified as a staff nurse in May 1986 and was employed on the special care baby unit (SCBU). Six months after starting, I was able to go to the John Radcliffe (JR) in Oxford to do the specialist course in Special and Intensive Care of the Newborn, which was very hard work, but I enjoyed it nevertheless.

I am sure that the stress caused to me by having Annie in the house was partly to blame for the return of my depression the following year. I had a friend, Cathy, who lived opposite – she and I did our neonatal intensive care course together on the John Radcliff unit – and she would sometimes call on Annie as a kind gesture. One day I met Cathy on the doorstep as she was coming out after visiting Annie. 'Veronica,' she said, 'I don't know how you can stand it!'

I spent some time benefiting from Hugh Wilson's wise counselling. I simply could not continue without someone to talk to and I realised that Hugh was the best person, although I had gone to the local church since we had moved to Chinnor. On one occasion he said seriously, 'Mother has *got* to go!' I could not find it in me to press the issue, however.

I would come home from work, drive into the garage and sit there trying to summon up the courage to go into the house to face Annie. As I entered the house she would say, 'Hello love,' in the most supremely pathetic manner. One day I came home and she was sitting halfway up the stairs. I asked her what was wrong. 'I felt all dizzy,' she told me.

'Where were you when you felt dizzy?' I asked.

'In the sitting room.'

'Well, why didn't you just sit down in the nearest chair and wait until it had gone off, like I told you to?'

'I just thought I had to get to my room.'

'Okay,' I said, 'just sit there until you feel better,' and went into the kitchen, closing the door. I did the washing-up – Annie would sit in the house all day and do nothing. When I went out into the hall again, Annie had somehow managed to get to her room. She did a similar thing to Richard – he sent for the doctor. He was genuinely worried about his mother.

One day Richard asked me if his mother should be referred to a specialist. I considered my answer carefully, then said, 'Your mother's problems are basically not physical.' I knew that Annie's problems were essentially psychological and that was the most tactful way I could put it. That was not to say that I thought there was nothing wrong with her. I had no doubt she was unhappy with her situation, and would rather have been living in her own home, but I also believed that she could have done much more to help herself. He was not happy with the answer I gave to his question, although he must have accepted it, as he did not mention the matter again. Annie's main problem was what health professionals call 'learned helplessness'.

Relations between me and Richard deteriorated. Richard would do nothing to support me in the care of his mother, indeed, he would often stay away from home all evening, or not even come home at all, yet he constantly criticised me for not being sympathetic enough to his mother. I can honestly say, however, that despite the strain she put me under, I never said a cross or unkind word to her. But, Richard would not stay home and look after his mother. I do not think that he could face that side of her.

Annie enrolled with a local GP. Despite my feeling that she was an adult and should be responsible for herself, I decided that I would have to talk to him myself. As soon as I sat down he said, 'This must be very difficult.' He wasn't joking.

The GP decided that once Annie had found somewhere to buy, she should spend a couple of weeks in the local cottage hospital 'to get her on her feet'. When the day came that she eventually left us and went into the hospital, I took her in. Richard went to work. I had been on nights for two weeks prior to Annie's entering the hospital. During that time I had been unable to cope with anything other than my work rota and, as a result, Annie simply took to her bed. She had not left her room for some days when I finished my night duty. That morning I went into her room and sat on the bed. I talked to her, telling her that staying in her room was doing her no good. I promising to take her out for a drive in the car if she would get up, get dressed and come out with me.

Annie's bed in the cottage hospital was upstairs and she made a great fuss of getting up the stairs, leaning on the arm of a nursing assistant. She refused to use the chairlift. The next day I could not bring myself to visit her; I was just relieved that she was someone else's problem. However, on the second day I went with Richard. When we arrived, Annie was downstairs chatting to the patients there. She came up, dressed and with make-up on, sat there and told us how nice the food was and how good the pastry was. I could have thrown their pastry at her. I had gone to such trouble while she was with us to get around her finickiness about food, searching the supermarkets for something she would eat. She would decide that she liked something, then invariably decided that she did not like it after all, further taxing my imagination. No way would she have eaten *my* pastry while she was with us.

When we got home, Richard and I had the inevitable argument. I was furious. As a nurse, I prided myself that I could tell the difference between real and conceived illness, yet even I had thought there was at least something wrong with Annie. But there she was, apparently fully recovered after two days in a cottage hospital. Richard argued that this was because the hospital had 'bucked her up'. He also told me that she had not eaten when she was with us because I had not provided 'sufficient variety'!

I wondered how it was that Richard was so blind that he could not see through his mother even then. Thinking about it afterwards, I decided that it was so obvious that Richard must have been able to see it. He was not arguing like he did despite his mother's miracle recovery, so much as because of it. Even faced with evidence, he could not bring himself to criticise her. It was as though fire and brimstone would be rained down on his head if he were found wanting where his mother was concerned.

I recovered slowly from Annie's stay and things began to go well. I enjoyed work as a staff nurse on the neonatal unit, spending the great majority of my time in the 'hot' nursery with the intensive-care babies, which I was quite competent to do following my course. I very much enjoyed the challenge. I was recognised as being the expert on technical matters and my colleagues, including the head of the electrical engineers department, would come to me for advice if there were any problems with the equipment. I always said that this was because I was the only one who ever read the manuals. I liked the responsibility of being in charge of the unit. One of my colleagues remarked, 'I like it when you're in charge. You're always so calm and unflappable, whatever the situation.' I also got on very well with the doctors. The junior doctors were usually quite happy to ask my advice. One time, however, a doctor ignored me until it got to the stage where I thought that it was becoming dangerous; enough for me to call the consultant to ask him to come to see the baby. The consultant came straight away and we had to take some drastic action to reverse the situation. He castigated the house officer for not having listened to me. When I was clearing up, I went into the clinical room where the consultant was talking to our senior nurse, Moira Campbell. As I came in, he commented to her, 'If it weren't for Veronica here, that baby would be dead by now.'

It was not that I expected the doctors to blindly follow my advice if they were in doubt – after all, they had to take the ultimate responsibility – but they could at least have got further advice if our views conflicted.

Everything seemed to be going well at work until the gradings were introduced in 1988. It was decided that nurses would be given a grade according to the work they did. I was the only staff nurse on the unit with the specialist qualification. The others were enrolled nurses who had done their specialist course, none of whom ever took charge, and specialist staff midwives. I was dismayed to learn that I had been graded with the enrolled nurses, despite their never taking the responsibility of being in charge of the unit as I did. The specialist staff midwives were all given the grade above me. I was further dismayed to see a piece of paper which supposedly justified my E grade. It said that I was not given credit for my neonatal qualification as I did not use it, and that I was never left in charge of the unit. These were both outright lies and the manager who had filled in the form knew that. I went to Moira, our senior nurse, in a fury. She crossed out the offending entries and gave it back to me, as if that would solve everything.

I was not the only one who was furious and upset as a result of their grade. The nursery nurses had been put on the same grade as the nursing assistants, with no recognition given to their childcare qualification. Their forms denied that they did babies' temperature, pulse and respirations – obs – although everyone knew that they were expected to do this as part of their routine. I was equally outraged on their behalf.

One of the nursery nurses, Alice, who was only just eighteen, had been advised by her union that she had a good case against her grade and should appeal. That being so, she went to Moira to tell her she would appeal. However, Moira bullied her into withdrawing, telling her that if she did appeal she would be moved onto the wards. As it happened there was a staff midwife in the office at the time. She was so appalled at Moira's attitude that she intervened on Alice's behalf. I saw this midwife later and asked her what had happened. Moira had always had the reputation of being very sweet and kind, but this midwife said, 'There'll be no more sweet Sister M for me!'

Always one to respond to an injustice, I was sufficiently fired up by all this to go to Moira myself to tell her that I would appeal. Although I had heard how she had treated Alice, I was still not prepared for the reaction I got. Moira told me that I would not be popular among certain people if I appealed, then tried to bribe me by reminding me of the sister's post about to come up. If she did but know it, this was just the sort of response calculated to make me all the more resolved. I told her that I did not expect to win my case – although the Royal College of Nursing (RCN) was supporting me, I had no faith in the system by then – but I was going to appeal anyway.

My appeal was heard on Wednesday, 8 February 1989.

There was a panel of three, led by the unit general manager, Dr Adams, with Mr Macey, a general manager. Helen Carter, a maternity manager, represented the staff side. I had an RCN representative with me, but she said nothing at all during the proceedings. She soon found out that I was quite capable of speaking for myself. From the way things went, I can only imagine that Mrs Carter expected the union representative, unfamiliar with the highly specialist SCBU, to speak for me while I said nothing.

Mrs Carter initiated with the statement 'Nurse Burton is a very inexperienced staff nurse and never takes charge without a senior member of staff being present.' She knew that these were blatant lies. I simply expressed my disagreement. There was a short discussion in which it was decided that the neonatal unit's off-duty would provide the answer.

Mrs Carter produced the off-duty, which was taken by Mr Macey, to my right. I asked him if I could see it and he passed it to me. One glance at it was sufficient to establish that my suspicions were correct. It was open on December, rather than closed and displaying January's rota. I handed it back. During December, Moira had taken to putting my name down as in charge when a unit charge nurse was on duty. She also did this for two other staff members – one a newly appointed charge nurse and another a staff midwife new to the unit. Although there may have been arguments for doing it with the latter two, I had never known it done before. I had gone to Moira and protested, saying that it was impossible for me to take charge properly when everyone inevitably went to the charge nurse. The result was that Moira told me I need not do it.

Dr Adams asked Mrs Carter if what she had produced was representative. She said it was. I stated that it was not.

At this point Mr Macey, who was examining the off-duty, said, 'Wait a minute, it says "in charge" next to Nurse Burton's name yet Moira Campbell was on.'

24

'Precisely,' I said.

Mrs Carter, choosing to ignore my remark, and presumably hoping that I would shut up, explained that this was a staff training exercise.

Given my chance to reply, I said, 'First, I was not told that and it seems to be a strange way to organise staff training when the purpose of the exercise has not been revealed to the member of staff concerned. Second, at the time I had asked why it was being done and was told that it was "to spread the load".' (Dr Adams commented that he had not realised that SCBU was so democratic.) 'Third, was December not a little late to train me to be in charge when I had been in charge, with no senior nurse present, for many months – as a further examination of the rota Mrs Carter had produced, would illustrate?'

At some point, Mrs Carter started to prevaricate. Mrs Carter would appear to be changing her argument; I thought, could we decide the point in question?

And so it went on. I was actually impressed by the way that Dr Adams conducted the appeal. At the end of it, I did at least establish that I was not inexperienced, that I did take charge on my own and that I did use my neonatal qualification. Their refusal to allow me the F grade was, I was told, because I was not in charge often enough. However, they based this on off-duty following the allocation of the gradings. The E grade had hurt my self-esteem to the extent that I told those who had previously been junior to me, and had been given an F grade, that they could take charge over me. Looking at the off-duty before the grading, as they should have done, it would have been evident that I was in charge often enough to qualify for the F grade. My RCN representative told me that I could take my appeal forward.

I went to Moira, told her that I had not won the appeal, but that I was still 'very angry at the way things have been done'.

It was now that Moira told me that I was one of her three best nurses, by far the most intelligent member of her nursing team, who could always be relied on to pick things up and put them right and who was a 'wizard with the machinery'. Why, in that case, had she not supported my appeal? I left her, not bothering to ask why she had written the off-duty so as to give Mrs Carter ammunition. Whose idea had that been?

I continued at work but my heart was no longer in it. My self-esteem had been badly affected by the grade I received. I had told Moira that I had been judged inferior to all those whom I would previously have considered my peers. The spectacle of my supposed superiors fabricating evidence and supporting their case with outright lies had left me deeply demoralised. I felt completely unappreciated in a job which I had previously enjoyed and found deeply fulfilling.

I continued to see Hugh at the rectory in High Wycombe. He recognised that I was becoming deeply depressed. Although I found him amazingly understanding, the message that I was becoming depressed again was something I found impossible to comprehend. Yet when I went to my GP complaining that I could not sleep, I told him that I had been depressed as a teenager. I could not understand myself.

The doctor said that, given my history, he thought that I should take antidepressants, but I refused them. I wanted nothing to do with the idea that I was becoming depressed again, and went away with nothing, although the doctor urged me to think about it. A few days later I made up my mind, almost in a state of panic. I had been on the late shift at work, and in charge. No intensive care cot was available since a radiant heater (a piece of equipment vital for giving medical and nursing care to a very ill baby) had been removed from the nursery for checking by the electronic engineers. Despite the fact that it had been passed safe for use, it had been left standing out in the corridor. It would take time to set up – time that we might not have if an emergency arrived, as it could do at any point. The sister on that morning had not got herself, or any of the other staff, organised and the unit was in chaos. Everyone on the late shift spent the entire time running around trying to do two things at once. I did not have a break and was still trying to attend to the paperwork, more important things having at last been done, when the night staff came on.

After report, Marcia, who was on that night, asked another of the nurses what was wrong. 'The morning staff did sod all, that's what's wrong!' she replied, as fed up as I was. I have to say that SCBU was usually run efficiently, which no doubt added to our exasperation.

I drove home feeling miserable, angry and frustrated, and taken for granted. It had been said that I did not take charge of the unit – too inexperienced, I was told – yet I was good enough to pick up the pieces after a charge nurse, if they did not happen to want to bother too much, I thought.

At that time anger usually turned into a sense of apathetic uselessness. There was no point in being angry. What did anyone care anyway? No one did, no one wanted to know. I felt primarily a sense of hopelessness and helplessness. I could not stand any more. I simply could not face it. Antidepressants? I was prepared at that moment to take anything that might help to relieve the pain, and it was pain I felt, as surely as if my leg had been crushed.

The next morning I telephoned the surgery and was told that my GP was at the main surgery, not at Chinnor. I was told that I would have to make an appointment to see him there if it was an emergency. I telephoned the other surgery and saw him in the little town nearby. He listened to me sympathetically and I left with a prescription for dothiepin hydrochloride (Prothiaden), an antidepressant.

That was in June, after which things had got worse rather than better. I still could not sleep – in fact, I wonder how I kept on my feet during the day as I had no more than two hours' broken sleep a night.

I kept going to work and somehow managed to do my job competently, but it was becoming an increasing strain.

My GP wrote me off work for a week 'to go and sit in the sun', of which there was plenty as the days of summer passed into the beginning of July. The doctor gave the cause of my illness as 'nervous debility'. Well, I thought, perhaps the rest would do me good. That's all I needed, a rest. I supposed that I was justified in taking the time off if the rest did some good. Good? What could be expected to do me good?

So there I was, after my week off, nothing having changed. I was getting hardly any sleep – how on earth did I keep going? There are few things worse than going to bed and knowing for certain that you will stay awake, hour after hour with your mind churning on and on – oh, why did it not stop? I thought. If only I could have some peace! I wanted some peace, some quiet, some rest, some SLEEP! My mind would not rest; it just went on and on and on. Was I going mad?

What have I done to deserve this? What have I done? – that was a silly question, for it was not really what I had done – there was no answer to that question. At least, it did not matter. It was nothing I had done, it was what I was, what I am – What else did I expect? I am useless, no good, I never did anything right – everything is going wrong and it is all my fault. Everything is my fault. They would all be better off without me, the whole world would be better off without me. I just make everything go wrong. It's all MY FAULT!

Alone, that is what I am. Alone – horribly, inevitably, on my own. No one can reach out to me, no one can touch me, no one can break through to me. I am alone, on my own, in total isolation.

So my thoughts went round and round, giving me nothing of comfort. In saner moments, I realised that Katherine and Nicholas had tried to help, always saying 'come and see us', 'stay for a meal'. They always made me welcome. It did not occur to me at the time that they realised something was wrong. How could they – there was nothing wrong, was there? If only I could . . .

I telephoned Hugh Wilson in High Wycombe, and went to see him. I talked to him, told him – well, I don't know what I told him but I talked a lot. In a way, it gave me a sense of relief. He told me that I was more depressed than my doctor thought and that I should go back to him and tell him more specifically how I felt. What he realised was that I was beginning to get serious suicidal feelings, and it was that that he thought I should clearly tell the GP 'otherwise they will just think that you are feeling sorry for yourself,' he commented.

I went back to the doctor. I told him that 'life is too much like hard work'. That was the closest I could get to that which Hugh felt I should say. It did not seem to have the right effect – but what was supposed to happen? I was not sure what I was supposed to do, what was supposed to happen. Somehow I felt that I had said the wrong things, or not said the right things, I did not know what. I felt that I had said the wrong things, somehow got it wrong. I did come away with something, though – a prescription for more antidepressants.

Monday, 10 July – it was almost two weeks since I had seen my GP – I had come home from an early shift and sat on my bed. I always sat on my bed. I felt awful, inexpressibly awful, my mind feeling paralysed, utterly without hope. I was so introspective that I could not get my thoughts together, get them to move away from the hopeless core and touch the world outside, respond to anything that was apart, around, beyond. There was nothing, nothing at all, no hope – none.

What could I do? What a ridiculous question. It was obvious. There was only one thing to be done. I got out my Data Sheet Compendium, with all the information it had about drugs. I looked up dothiepin hydrochloride, the antidepressant I was taking. It said:

> The smallest dose of Prothiaden alone which resulted in the death of an adult was reported to be 0.75–1.0 g. The largest dose from which recovery took place was reported to be 5.0 g.

There it was, all I needed to know. I took my tablets, tipped them out, and counted them. I had a good idea of how much of the drug I had in total. I usually did, as I often counted them out. I had done that with my drugs when I was a teenager. When nothing else provided anything of worth, knowing you had enough of the drug to destroy yourself was the only comfort to be had.

I did not have a lot, but there was the prescription. I looked at it, calculated the dosage and added it to what I already had. In all,

I had more than 1 gram but less than 5 grams. A lot depended, though, on the circumstances. My weight was not much, especially since I had been steadily losing weight – I was living on little more than biscuits and drinking chocolate made in the microwave. I should not need as much as 5 grams, but then I had to be sure, I could not risk getting it wrong. One important point, though, was that I was not likely to be found until the drug had had plenty of time to get into my system. I knew that Richard would not look into my room either that evening when he came home, or the next morning before leaving for work. I was on a late shift the next day, due on at 13.30. By the time anyone at work decided to investigate my failure to arrive, Richard would be at work and they only had my home telephone number. By then, hopefully, I would be beyond hearing the telephone.

It is often assumed that if someone kills themselves, or seriously considers doing so, they are so out of their mind that they do not know what they are doing. If only it were that simple. My thoughts began turning around in my head once again. They had to start churning around and taking me away from that state of decisiveness. I was horrified, scared. But why was I always so weak? I thought. Will I never get myself out of this? I think the answer must be no – that is awful, that is real hopelessness. I can only think of one thing worse. What if you had done everything you could have done to ensure that they could not bring you back, and yet they managed to? To wake up when you had thought never to wake again? I thought of that man on my night duty as a student nurse.

I remembered doing my accident and emergency experience as a student. I had been surprised, and actually quite angered, by the attitude of the staff to patients who had taken an overdose. It had invariably been assumed that the person's action was a dramatic and hysterical act that resulted in a waste of nursing and medical time that could have been devoted to those who were really ill, and through no fault of their own. Of course, anyone who performs a suicidal act but survives, or is prevented from getting so far as to act, is always open to the charge that it was not their real intent at all.

Could I be quite sure that I had enough drugs to kill me? I would have to wait, I decided, until I was able to get my prescription. The reason I did not take my tablets was, in part, because I did not have the means immediately available – I would need to go to the chemist to get the prescription made up.

Maybe it was also symptomatic of my usual diurnal variation in mood. As the time passed towards evening, I began to think more clearly, became aware of how terrifyingly irrevocable the act would be.

I went through a stage of feeling anxious – anxious and vacillating. The idea that there was a choice, something that had seemed not to exist, made me confused and uncertain. What should I do? What was going on? I did not understand. Yet a few hours ago I had had it all sorted out, hadn't I?

I picked up the receiver from the telephone by the bed. I telephoned Wycombe Rectory. Hugh was in. I cannot remember what I said, but he commented that I was very distressed, he could tell from my voice. He told me to put the telephone down and stay where I was; he would telephone my GP. When he phoned back, he told me that he had spoken to one of the other partners, as my GP was away. Hugh told me to see that doctor, or another in the practice, as soon as possible.

When I telephoned, the receptionist responded as soon as I gave my name, and told me to come about midday. I entered the surgery to find it quite empty, and was told to go through to the doctor straight away. It did not occur to me until sometime after, that midday was outside normal surgery hours.

I went in to see the doctor, the one whom Hugh had spoken to. He was the senior doctor in the practice. He spent some time listening to me, and responded sympathetically. 'Your vicar friend says that you are suicidal. Is that true?' I remembered how Hugh had told me to be precise, to say how I was really feeling, yet I could not bring myself to answer the question outright.

'You're not denying it,' the doctor observed.

I shook my head. I could not deny it.

He suggested that he could keep writing me off sick until I found another job elsewhere, or he could refer me to a psychiatrist. I did not give him a decision, I could not decide on anything. He then decided for himself that he would refer me. He asked me where I wished to be referred – presumably not High Wycombe – Aylesbury or Oxford? Again I could not make a decision so it was made for me. He decided to send me to Oxford.

Meanwhile, I returned to work, where Moira continued with the negative view of me put forward in the appeal.

Chapter 4 ▬▬

One thing that made Moira's new attitude particularly hard to cope with was that previously my view had always been listened to with respect and my suggestions followed. On one shift, before the gradings were ever thought of, I was the nurse in charge of the unit when a midwife rushed in from the labour ward with a baby she reported to have gone blue. The baby had regained colour by then but the midwife explained that the parents had called urgently and she could see that the baby was very cyanosed. I helped the nurse and the doctor to stabilise the little girl, then left her in the hands of the doctor and allocated nurse to go to talk to the parents. The doctor looked up and said, 'Tell them she's all right, we're just doing some tests.'

'I can't do that,' I protested. I learned a lot from Jenni, our bereavement councellor, while I was working on SCBU, having taken a particular interest in using counselling skills with parents whose baby was dead or abnormal in some way. You always told the truth.

I went to the parents, first asking them what they had seen. The

31

mother described how her little daughter had gone blue in her arms and her husband had shouted for help. The midwife grabbed the baby and rushed to the special care unit with her. Clearly the parents had seen enough to cause them great concern. To pass it off as something that could be solved by doing a few tests would obviously be quite untenable. Everyone has heard about 'blue babies' and in most people's minds it means a heart problem. I therefore explained that we did not know what was wrong as yet, but we would keep them in touch with the situation and would explain everything fully and truthfully. I answered their questions then returned to the unit. It is important to make contact with the parents to reassure them that everything is being done for their baby and that the staff of SCBU are concerned for them. It also helps with the establishment of the parents' relationship with their baby early on, something that is vitally important for all parents and babies and which can be disrupted by early problems if they are not managed carefully.

I went back to SCBU, where the nurse and doctor were still involved with the baby from labour ward. I explained what I had said. The doctor looked at me disapprovingly, so I said, 'What if we have to send her to Oxford under a blue light?'

'Oh, I don't think it will come to that,' she answered.

As things turned out she was not sent to Oxford in an emergency ambulance, but to Great Ormond Street (GOS), so it was just as well I had prepared the parents for the possibility of a serious condition. The good thing was that the baby's condition was such that, when GOS operated they would be able to correct the abnormality, which allowed fluids and food to go down her trachea (windpipe), blocking it and causing the cyanosis. Once given a successful surgical repair, she would be without problems from it for the rest of her life. One of my own sisters had the same problem but has had no difficulties from it since she was operated on.

The next day I told Moira what I had done and she endorsed my decision to be honest with the parents.

There was no shortage of money on SCBU, as it was not unusual for a person to come to the unit door to give over a cheque for hundreds of pounds, explaining that they had made some sponsored effort and had decided to give the proceeds to SCBU. Ill babies or children easily attracted people's generosity. I often felt like pointing out that there was a ward for the elderly on the other side of the hospital, which would be delighted to receive some money to get decent chairs for the patients, or some such thing. It was seldom sponsor money was contributed to that ward, despite its being in great need of finance. SCBU, however, was continually receiving gifts. It allowed us to buy the most up-to-date equipment. One day we received £8000 worth of the latest monitoring equipment. Apart from monitoring temperature, respiration and heart rate, it also subcutaneously (through the skin) measured pO_2 (partial pressure of oxygen – the level of oxygen in the blood) and pCO_2 (the level of carbon dioxide). It was the first time we had equipment capable of measuring subcutaneous pCO_2, which was more problematic than measuring subcutaneous oxygen levels, and that means of measuring carbon dioxide was quite new.

Despite the fact that the equipment was brand new, nurses were repeatedly complaining of its not working and calling the electrical engineers department. I used it one evening and found nothing wrong but the next morning it was outside the nursery with a note saying that it was malfunctioning. Ray, the head of the engineers department came to me, as he often did when a nurse complained of equipment malfunction. 'Veronica, what's wrong with the new monitor?' he asked.

'As far as I'm concerned – nothing,' I replied. He took the monitor down to his department and sought me out when he returned it to the unit. He said he could find nothing wrong with it.

The fact remained, however, that nurses were still not satisfied and I felt that there had to be some explanation. On a quiet day, therefore, I sat with the monitor in front of me and the manual in my hands. I read systematically through the manual. Eventually I came to what I was sure was the solution, in a chapter describing the technicalities of pCO_2 monitoring. I went to Moira, in the office, and told her I thought I had the solution to the problems that nurses were having with the new equipment and that I would go down to Ray to tell him. He understood when I explained it to him, and even produced a booklet on the subject, lending it to me. The solution was to programme the monitor to make adjustments; without that, the figure for carbon dioxide levels appeared to be way out of the normal range. This was what led the staff to complain that it was not working.

A couple of days later, I was caring for a baby with whom we were using the new monitor. The consultant stopped on his round to ask how it was functioning. I said that it was fine. He then noticed the red 'A' for adjustment next to the pCO_2 reading and asked what it meant. I explained the basis of the carbon dioxide monitoring and why I used it that way. This led to a discussion between me and the consultant, with him feeling that we should not use the adjustment function. This went on until someone reminded us that there was supposed to be a consultant's round taking place.

Later that morning Moira beckoned me into the office. She asked what the consultant and I had been discussing and why I was disagreeing with him. I therefore started to explain from the beginning, the nature of pCO_2 monitoring. She interrupted me, saying, 'Oh, I don't understand all that. We'll do it your way.' Later, the other consultant agreed with me so it was decided to use the adjustment facility.

This was all before the grading. Moira could hardly avoid the fact that I was competent at my job and that that I was respected by other professionals involved in the running of SCBU. I continued to work after I had received my grading and no one picked me up on any errors.

We had once put out a fast bleep as my baby's tracheal tube (which should be positioned such as to deliver respiratory gases – air and oxygen – to the lungs) had shifted from its proper position. The doctor who came had not yet intubated (placed a new tube in the right position) a baby in an emergency and looked horrified when she realised the situation. I said that the situation was under control, and she could take her time. I had been taught to intubate on my neonatal course at the John Radcliffe but did not get the practice at Wycombe to maintain my skills. After I had received my grading and stated that I was considering leaving, this doctor, who was about to move from her first six months on SCBU as a junior house officer and to start her last six months as a senior house officer, said, 'Don't leave until I've finished my senior post.'

From the time I received my grading, I became increasingly demoralised. It was a process accelerated by the grading appeal that I attended. Although I made no serious errors (or, indeed, any errors at all that anyone else picked up) – which was incredible in itself – my tolerance levels were, however, beginning to diminish. I was normally a very patient person but I found myself needing to make an increasing effort to keep my temper or to hold my irritation. Amazingly, I went on working until two days before I was admitted to hospital but I knew that, although I seemed to continue functioning at a high level, I was finding it hard to tolerate others' shortcomings.

The last shift I did before I went to outpatients was a late shift, 13.30–21.30. I was on with Dianne, who was in charge that evening. I was caring for a baby on constant positive airways pressure (CPAP), with the plan being to extubate him (remove the tracheal tube and leave him to breathe on his own) later that evening. However, his pCO_2 was so unstable that it was being suggested that the baby might need to be put back on intermittent positive pressure ventilation (IPPV), where the ventilator did the entire work of breathing for him. I looked at the blood gas chart and established that the new monitor had been reading remarkably accurately all day. I also investigated the carbon dioxide level and discovered that it had been rising steadily all day without anyone apparently feeling the need to intervene. Now they planned to take the extreme measure of returning the baby to full-scale respiratory support. Ventilation saves lives, but inevitably it can cause complications. No baby should be ventilated unless absolutely necessary, and never for longer than necessary.

I reached for the stethoscope, whereupon Debbie, the doctor, commented, 'He sounded quite clear this morning.' I just managed, with unusual difficulty, to answer that. What had been the case on the round at nine o'clock that morning was past history at half-past three that afternoon, especially in the case of a sick neonate. I was severely tempted to say something sharp to that effect, but I managed to avoid it. Despite Moira's criticisms, I don't think that I have ever made a bad-tempered remark to anyone, though by the time this event occurred I had to make a conscious effort to avoid it. Hearing the baby's chest, it was obvious that he was drowning in his own secretions and that this was the most obvious cause of his rising pCO_2. Despite all the necessary information being there, neither the nurse nor the doctor caring for him had done anything about the situation. I remembered the jibe made at my grading appeal, that I was an 'inexperienced staff nurse' – but not so inexperienced that I could not pick up the pieces after others' errors, I thought bitterly. I was not normally one to think like this but my increasing depression was making me far less tolerant than I would normally have been. Normally I would have felt some irritation but would have dismissed it as the way things went at times.

I told Debbie that I thought the baby had a problem with secretions and the best course of action would be to give regular suction and physiotherapy, to clear the secretions, while the baby remained on CPAP, and thereby hopefully to avoid the necessity of switching back to IPPV. The doctor accepted this.

During the shift I managed to get the pCO_2 onto a downward trend, but it was not as smooth a trend as I would have liked. When the doctor came to review the situation, we discussed it and I gave my view that it would be best to keep the baby on CPAP until the morning, then consider extubation. One of our consultants was sitting at the desk outside the nursery. The doctor went and relayed what I had said. The consultant looked through the glass at me and put up her thumb to convey that she agreed with me.

Having had that endorsement I began to feel better, however, a baby was brought from the labour ward at about 20.30. She was a good-sized term baby who had experienced a difficult birth and had shown signs of asphyxia. It was the sort of baby best left alone to recover of her own accord. The doctor on call, however, decided to do blood gases by means of an arterial stab, so called because you had to take a needle and stab it down and through to the artery – deeper than the veins from which normal blood samples are usually taken. It is essential to use arterial blood for blood gas analysis. The usual way to do this in a neonate was to place a cannula through an artery in the umbilical cord, thereby making it possible to take arterial blood samples painlessly. This baby, however, did not have an umbilical catheter.

When the doctor said that she was going to do an arterial stab, I asked why. 'To see how asphyxiated it is,' she answered. Once again having to repress my irritation, I pointed out that the baby was now pink and her observations were normal. That being so, was it necessary to subject her to the trauma of an arterial stab? The doctor refused to listen, so I walked out of the nursery to avoid saying anything that I would regret. Dianne appeared at that moment and I described to her what was happening. She went in and remonstrated with the doctor, but to no avail.

I felt a rising sense of frustration and anger. I objected to pain being inflicted on a baby for no good reason, as it seemed to me was happening. Apart from that, the doctor failed to do a successful arterial stab and therefore distressed the baby quite unnecessarily.

I went home to an empty house, feeling quite awful that night. The next morning I could not face work. I had gone on working all that time since I had first received the shock of an E grade, but finally I had to admit defeat.

Chapter 5 ▄▄▄

Psychiatric outpatient appointment – Admission to Phoenix

July 1989 was sunny and hot, as indeed was the rest of that long summer. It was only eight o'clock yet it was already warm as I drove my car into the cul-de-sac and drew to a halt. The appointment was not until a quarter to nine and the hospital was only a couple of minutes' drive away but I had been anxious to be there on time and had got up far too early – but then, I had not slept all night so it made little difference how early I got up.

Half an hour later I drove into the hospital and stopped outside the outpatients department, separate from the edifice of the old county asylum. I kept my eyes to the ground and did not even glance at it.

I could already feel the warmth of the sun as I got out of the car but it made no impression on me. I had always loved the sunshine; as a child I would always be a deep tanned colour from spending long periods in the sun. Despite the heat, I did not experience any pleasure that day. I had become immune to it, not only on that day but also weeks, even months before. Long after, I would remember that day in its detail – no, not simply remember that day but in a sense I would never stop *feeling* it. I can vividly recall the hot sun, the unfamiliarity, fear even, confusion, vulnerability.

I went in and presented myself to the receptionist, who was surprised. She said that she had received a message to say that I would not be coming for my appointment. I was equally surprised as I had telephoned to confirm my attendance as requested. The person I had spoken to must have got it wrong. Not surprising, perhaps, especially given the quietness with which I had come to speak at that time. Presumably I had been misheard. The receptionist assured me that I would be seen. The concern with which she did this surprised me – why should it matter anyway? Surely it did not matter to the receptionist or to anyone else, including me.

I went into the waiting room as directed. I took a quick, carefully disguised look around. There was a young woman in a leather jacket accompanied by someone I took to be her mother. An odd thing to notice, given that the room was full of people I was hardly aware of. There she was. Accompanied. I was alone. I felt the room was full of strangers, which made me feel threatened and self-conscious.

The letter I had received giving me the appointment had also asked that I bring a friend or relative with me. It further said that a doctor or social worker might interview them and that they should be prepared to be at the hospital for one to two hours. The obvious person to go with me was Richard, but we had not spoken for several weeks. Richard had contracted ringworm so I had started to sleep in the spare room (I could not risk catching it given that I worked with tiny babies on the special care baby unit). As I became increasingly depressed, Richard had spent more and more time out of the house, even spending nights away. I wondered why he had to work so hard just when I most needed him. It was very odd. In retrospect, perhaps, it was because I needed him, and because of how much I needed him.

On receiving the letter, I had wondered what I should do about it. I hoped that Richard would go with me but decided that it would be best not to approach him directly. Instead I left the letter for him to read. He came in late, as usual. I waited until he had had plenty of time to read the letter then went downstairs. That was when I brought up the subject of the appointment.

Richard said that he had not been asked to read the letter, 'but as it happens, I have'. I felt that this was somewhat disingenuous. I knew that he would read the letter when I had put it there – there was never really any doubt that he would. He went on to say, 'And if you think I'm going to be interviewed for hours by a doctor or social worker . . .'

It was really no more than I had expected – Richard had not been speaking to me for some time, but I was nevertheless distressed by his refusal. It was quite tragic that our relationship had reached such a low point. One of the things that had attracted me to Richard was his sense of humour. I remembered when his mother had got a little dog and called him Robbie. One day the dog was suffering from diarrhoea. 'Poor thing,' his mother said, 'Little Robbie, Robbie the Bruce.'

'More like Robbie the Loose,' Richard immediately responded. It was his sense of humour that had attracted me to him. There was no humour in our relationship by then.

I went to bed, curled up and cried and cried. When I stopped crying, all those awful thoughts came back to my mind, unsought and uninvited, and those horrible thoughts circled unceasingly in my head. When I am depressed, my thoughts are quite different from those that are in my head when I am sane and clear-headed. Also, I seem incapable of challenging them in any way, or dismissing them, as I would normally do. Everything is extreme, in a manner impossible for most people to imagine. When depressed, you can never imagine something positive occurring, such as an improvement in your profoundly distressed state. Your mind tells you that that *will not* happen, that it is *not possible* and you *know* it, firmly and irrevocably. There is nothing to be gained from simply contradicting someone in this state, for it will simply cause further distress and reinforce their sense that they exist apart from all around them. Even if someone has never suffered extreme pain, they will know what pain is like and can extrapolate reasonably successfully, so that they can feel sympathy for someone who rolls around the bed in agony. It can, however, be impossible for a person to appreciate the extreme distress caused by the thoughts of a deeply depressed person. I was unable to see myself as worthy or useful in any way. My thoughts constantly persecuted me and I felt real *pain*. It is impossible for some people to imagine the reality of extreme psychological pain, accepting as they are willing to, the phenomenon of extreme physical pain.

I hardly slept all night and, as the time approached for the alarm clock to go off, I felt so awful that I wondered if I could face work at all that day. For the first time since all these troubles had started, I contemplated taking the day off work. But it did not seem right to do so when there was nothing really wrong with me. I got up and walked into the bathroom and looked in the mirror – one look at my face, eyes dark-rimmed, puffy and red – and I knew that I could not walk into the unit looking like that. In the bedroom I picked up the telephone and rang the hospital, asking for the bleep carrier for the maternity unit. I did not recognise the voice of the person who answered. I first asked how many were on SCBU that morning. I explained that I did not feel well and thought I might not come in that day. 'Never mind how many are on the unit,' the voice answered emphatically, 'you do not sound at all well and should stay at home.' Another oddity, I thought, that I should sound ill when there was nothing wrong with me. What was going on? What was happening with my life?

That day I hardly moved from the bed. Richard went to work then came home again without, as usual, looking into the spare room. I had counted up my tablets and considered it often enough recently. Did he care?

Once again I had a bad night. So I had dressed early and gone to the hospital – Thursday, 20 July 1989 – I always remember that date.

In the waiting room I went straight for the only empty chair that my quick scan of the room had revealed. I sat down and curled up, keeping my eyes fixed closely onto the hands which I constantly wrung together in my lap.

'Veronica Burton,' someone called. At the sound of my name I got up and walked to the open door, still wringing my hands and keeping my head down, looking only at the floor. I stood in front of the person in the corridor but I did not look up. He introduced himself as Dr Andrews, a senior registrar, then explained that, if I did not object, I would be interviewed for an hour by a medical student, after which they would discuss my case, then see me together. I did not object. I would do what I was told as I did not care anyway. The medical student was introduced as Stephen. I followed him into an interview room. He sat at the table with a set of notes in which he wrote as the interview progressed. I sat, as requested, in the chair beside the desk. I curled up and watched myself wringing my hands as I had in the waiting room. Stephen had to lean forward to hear my almost-whispered answers. He asked questions about my family, about my previous experience of depression when a teenager, about work, Richard and home, about how I felt. Dr Andrews looked in, presumably after an hour, but Stephen asked for more time. After another fifteen minutes or so, the first interview ended and I returned to my seat in the waiting room.

I do not know how long I sat there before Dr Andrews returned and asked me to sit in the interview room again. The medical student was there but this time it was Dr Andrews who spoke to me. I was not aware of how long this interview lasted or when it was that the suggestion was made that I go into hospital. I was stunned, unable to react. It all seemed very unreal. Did he really mean me? Me – Veronica – to go into hospital? But there was nothing wrong with me. Of course he did not mean it, it was not real.

'You won't need to go home and get anything – we can provide what you need, can't we?' he said. I wondered why he said that. Why shouldn't I go home?

One thing that did impress me was the sensitive manner in which he dealt with the situation. It was not, 'Oh help! This is a disastrous situation – we had better take drastic measures!' but, 'You have suffered with this long enough' and 'You need to be somewhere where you will be looked after.'

Dr Andrews asked me if I would let him make arrangements for my admission. I could not respond. I simply sat, leant forwards, looking at the floor. I did not say yes, I did not say no. I simply sat looking at the floor.

The doctor sat patiently awaiting an answer. I began to feel that I should give an answer and that the answer should be 'no' but I could not say it. I felt confused. Here was someone approaching me with kindness and gentleness, someone who understood that I was suffering – and who seemed to believe that I deserved help. He told me that I was ill, that I should be in hospital. Dr Andrews had referred to the confusion as to whether or not I would keep the appointment, and had remarked twice, 'I'm glad you did come.' It was very odd. Why should anyone be glad at my coming? Why should anyone think that I deserved help?

I was so amazed and confused that I could not reply. I did not know what to do or say.

Dr Andrews leaned forward and said, 'I'll go and arrange it, shall I?'

Still I said nothing. Dr Andrews decided to take this as assent. He touched me lightly on the arm, then stood up and left the room, leaving me with the medical student. It was strange how effective that brief touch was. Its effect was out of all proportion to the amount of physical contact it allowed. Here was someone who was not intent on keeping his distance, on preserving my separateness, on colluding with me in maintaining my isolation – someone who knew something of what I felt, what I thought – what I was. He had reached out and touched me. I had thought myself untouchable.

In the meantime Stephen made a courageous attempt to keep up some form of conversation. Throughout the day I was surprised at his consistent willingness to talk to me as if I were an intelligent individual, despite my uncommunicative state. Not only did he insist on speaking to me much longer, I suspect, than many people would have done, but he spoke on subjects that would normally have interested me. I remember that he asked me which of Mahler's symphonies I most liked. I was glad he did not speak to me as if I were stupid, even though I was acting as if I were.

Dr Andrews eventually returned and, taking the trouble to sit down and lean forwards to speak to me quietly, he explained that there were problems finding me a bed, which meant that I would have to go to a different ward than the one to which I would otherwise have gone. This worried me and I asked where I would go. Dr Andrews assured me that I would still be in the same hospital. He went away again.

Why hadn't I told him not to bother? If there were problems finding a bed, I would go home. There was no need to worry about it; I did not want a bed anyway. Why hadn't I said that? I could not say it, yet I could not understand why. Why had I not told him and gone away? Gone home. I could not understand why I did not say it; it seemed the obvious solution. Perhaps even then I was getting signals that I would not be allowed to go. He had told me that I could not go home to get my belongings.

On his second return he again apologised for the delay and suggested that it would be better if we went over to the main hospital where I could sit in the waiting room. Outside the sun shone brightly. For long after it still saddened me how unresponsive I had been to the beautiful weather, the sort of weather that came so rarely and which I normally enjoyed.

As we walked across the grass, Dr Andrews told me that it looked like I would be on Dr Nick Rose's unit. He asked me if I knew him, as he had worked in the same hospital as I had before he moved to Oxford. I shook my head in reply.

Inside the main door of the hospital we went to the left and entered the waiting room. Dr Andrews advised caution, as some of the chairs were not particularly safe. The room was large, with big sash windows, a table in the centre and a big red carpet. I took this in in one carefully disguised glance. It was dangerous to look up, someone might meet your look and that was a challenge I felt unable to cope with.

There were some magazines somewhere – I could not remember where – and Stephen offered me one, which I refused. He looked at one himself and made the occasional comment to me. He had stayed when Dr Andrews went away again. It seemed that I was not to be left alone. Seeing the relevant part of my notes much later, I discovered that Dr Andrews suggested the use of the Mental Health Act if I tried to leave. He also noted that I had agreed to be admitted 'reluctantly'.

I actually discovered from my notes generally that a section had been suggested far more often than I was aware of, if my behaviour – such as insisting that I go home – warranted it. (Application of the Mental Health Act, a section of which can be used to detain a patient in hospital and/or treat them without their consent, if their mind is so disturbed that they are held unable to make rational judgements.) I could have been on a section a number of times if I had been even more uncooperative than I often was. Sometimes I knew that there was a chance of putting me on a section and deliberately avoided acting in such a way as to bring it about. I could only think that way, however, when I was not severely depressed; then I simply lacked the initiative to move from my room.

Dr Andrews returned to tell us that he had ordered some lunch for us. Until then I had not thought about what time of the day it was. I had not looked at my watch all morning. Before Dr Andrews left again he went over and said something to me, I cannot remember what, and touched me on the arm again, that light, sensitive touch.

Sandwiches, two yoghurts and some fruit were brought in for our lunch with two cups of tea. I did not feel hungry, but neither did I feel like bothering to refuse, so I ate what I was offered.

It must have been late afternoon when we finally left that room. I cannot remember when I realised that we were waiting for transport to take us to another hospital, which I had never heard of. When I did realise, I became anxious lest I be separated from the two people who had come to represent some degree of security to me, however tenuous. I had recognised Stephen's attempts to put me at my ease and was grateful for it. I realised, though, that it was the doctor who would have the real influence to exert. I asked Stephen, in a very rare attempt at unsolicited speech, whether Dr Andrews worked at the other hospital. Stephen was not sure, but he thought not. My anxiety about the situation increased. I asked where the hospital was but all that Stephen could say was that he thought it was somewhere around the ring road.

All this time my car had been sitting outside the outpatients building. I remembered that I had left my car sunroof open. Stephen said that we could go and close it and accompanied me out of the building and over to the car. I thought fleetingly of getting in the car and driving away, but I did not have the energy for stunts like that. I then realised that what I most wanted was safety, security, hence my dismay when I realised that I was to be taken away from Stephen and Dr Andrews, and taken I did not know where, and left in the care of I did not know who. I wondered if I would have felt less disorientated and confused if I had had someone I knew with me. I felt very alone and unprotected.

The problem, so it appeared, was in getting an ambulance to take me to the other hospital. The problem was eventually solved when a nurse manager, whose name I forgot almost as soon as he introduced himself, came in and told me that he would take me in his own car to save waiting any longer. He apologised for the wait and assured me that it was not the way they usually did things. I wondered why he apologised. It did not matter to me if I waited, or indeed where I waited. Nothing mattered, really.

Dr Andrews had expressed his concern at my having driven to the hospital. 'People who feel like you sometimes feel tempted to . . .'

'Drive into a tree,' I completed for him.

He nodded, looking serious. Later he expressed the same concern.

The nurse manager mentioned my car, saying that it would be safer parked nearer the hospital. He suggested that I gave him the key so that he could move it. I said that I could move it. He answered that of course I could, but he would be quite happy to do it for me. I handed him my keys. Although he was apparently amenable to my suggestion, I had the feeling that I did not, in reality, have a choice. The car was moved and locked, and the key was put in an envelope and left at reception for Richard to collect. We then set off for the other hospital. I sat in the back, with Stephen in the front passenger seat. On the way, he and the manager discussed the shortage of nursing staff. Stephen remarked that the exams on psychiatry he had to pass were much easier than those the nursing students had to do.

I sat and stared out of the window. I was driven through backstreets that I did not recognise, so I felt quite disorientated when we finally arrived at the hospital.

The impression I got of Littlemore Hospital was, at that point, very vague. We went through what appeared to be a side entrance – a door kept open with a mat put across the doorstep. Inside there was a low table and some chairs. I was asked to wait there with Stephen. I was not to be left alone for a minute.

The manager returned with Tim Woodward, whom he introduced as a charge nurse. I later got it into my head that his name was Tim, but at that moment I forgot it as soon as I was told it. The manager then left, apologising once more for the delay. Stephen said goodbye and wished me luck. The whole situation left me feeling abandoned, confused and disorientated. It had been a long, bright, hot day, which in itself accentuated the dark, restricted isolation of my mind. I knew the centre of the city, but once taken out of that area I was no longer able to keep my bearings. My awareness of my surroundings was greatly limited by my reluctance, or inability, to raise my eyes from the ground. This also made it difficult for me to keep any form of mental picture of the people to whom I was introduced; that, and my confused state of mind, made it difficult for me to keep names in my head.

I was able to absorb neither faces nor names into my mind.

Tim took me through what seemed to be an immense hall, high-ceilinged with large sash windows. We went into the kitchen, smaller in all senses than the room we had just come through. He told me that the kitchen had recently been refitted – perhaps because this was his excuse for not knowing where the cups were. He laughed, saying that he did not know where anything was now, to some other person who was in the kitchen.

We went to sit in the 'quadrangle', a square room that was rather scruffy (as, it has to be said, was the rest of the Phoenix ward). Once again I got a sense of immensity, with those high ceilings and windows. I became aware that the quad was some sort of social centre for the ward. At some point I was put into the care of Amanda, a student nurse. Amanda was with me when Claire, a registrar, came to see me. I never saw her again; she was presumably the registrar on call.

The interview started in the quad, but we moved into the 'blue room' as another patient came into the quadrangle and did something of which I was only dimly aware (as usual I was sitting with my head down, looking at the floor) – I thought he had vomited.

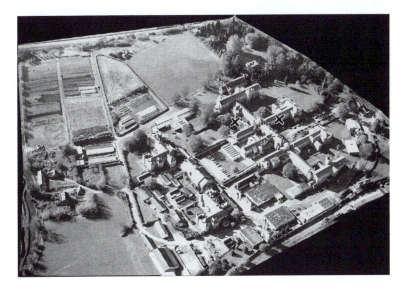

Figure 5.1 The old Littlemore Hospital from the air, showing the extent of the grounds. The first cross shows the side entrance through which I originally entered the hospital. The second shows the courtyard, with its great trees, that I liked to walk around and to which I so often looked when confined inside.

45

'Oh, Alan!' Claire said despairingly, and then suggested that we go through to the blue room. This room was also large, but for the first time there was a carpet underfoot, blue and green – not colours that I would have chosen to put together. Who was responsible for that?

I was asked the same sort of questions that I had been asked at outpatients. Dr Andrews had asked me if I had lost weight, saying that I looked very thin. This was followed by the inevitable question as to whether I knew how much I had lost, to which I shook my head. In fact, I did know but it was still a sensitive issue for me and it felt safer to simply deny that I knew. The same questions I had answered earlier that day came from Claire, and she received the same responses. It was, though, the depression that caused the weight loss.

After the medical interview was over, there were still the nursing notes to go through. Tim reappeared at this point, explaining to Amanda what needed to be done. She had to write a description of me. I wondered if this was in case I escaped? – this idea added to the unreality of the situation. I had a glimpse of myself running away, pursued by the nurses. It seemed quite absurd, yet I was later to discover that it was not quite such an unlikely event as I thought. Amanda asked if I had anything valuable with me. I answered that I had some money and my credit cards. Amanda said that she would get an envelope for them and have them put into the safe. She must have forgotten, however, and I did not remind her as the thought occurred to me that I would need them if I was going to get away from that place. That I was to stay there was a fact that I had yet to come to terms with.

We went outside, Amanda remaining with me. We sat down by a large lawn, though we did not stay out for long. Amanda did all the talking, telling me that she was an enrolled nurse doing a conversion course. Being myself a nurse, this meant something to me and helped me to remember Amanda. She also told me that she lived in a village, the name of which I recognised as being one where Richard and I had once looked at a house. All these facts acted like mental hooks on which to secure the picture of Amanda that I was building up in my mind. A name on its own was no use. Since I was unable to look anyone in the face, I had no idea of how they looked physically. I was very reliant on what was said. Sometimes something would happen while I was with someone that would help me to remember them. Tim was introduced as a charge nurse; he was the first member of staff I had met; he did not know where the cups were in the kitchen. Amanda was with me when I first saw a doctor; she filled in the information sheet for my nursing file; she told me a couple of things about herself that I remembered.

There was another person in the kitchen when I was there with Tim. I knew this because Tim spoke to him, but I had not the faintest idea of who it was or what he was doing.

Whenever a nurse was introduced, only their name was given. In other circumstances, this may have sufficed. But as things were, a name alone was hopelessly inadequate. Looking back, it seemed peculiar to me how difficult I found it to distinguish one person from another. All the staff later came to have their own identities. Initially, however, I found it all very confusing. Not even a title – staff nurse, nursing assistant etc. – was used. It was explained to me that this was because each person was a member of a team in which they each had equal importance. That I basically agreed with, but I failed to see how using a title detracted from it. Maybe it was because I was a nurse myself that the use of the titles would have been helpful to me, would have helped me to identify individuals, but they were never used as it was felt that that was not in keeping with the nurses' sense of equality within the team. I rather wished that they would have put aside that particular principle in order to give me just that little bit more by which to remember them as individuals. Tim and Amanda, the two nurses I had met that day, I remembered (although I did not actually meet Amanda again – she must have gone to another ward).

I went through that first day feeling an increasing degree of disorientation, confusion and bewilderment. I had been moved from the hospital that I could at least locate, to I did not know where. I had come to have a tenuous sense of security in the two persons who had dealt with me from the beginning, only to be separated from them and put in the care of total strangers. In retrospect, I realised how good the nurses were. At the time, however, the unfamiliarity of everything and everyone around me made the whole situation seem threatening. There was no stability, no familiarity, no recognition – everything had changed, I was on my own and had lost all control of my environment.

I was told that if I wanted to telephone anyone, I could use the office phone. I telephoned Richard to say that I had been admitted to hospital and would not be home that day. Richard did little more than acknowledge having understood. I also telephoned Hugh Wilson. He was not surprised when I said I had been admitted.

Chapter 6

First night in Phoenix – Consultant's visit – Richard's first visit – Close observation – I leave unit and am brought back

The evening of my arrival at Phoenix ward, Karen, another of the ward charge nurses, took me to my room and made up the bed for me. The room was at the far end of a corridor that opened onto the quad. It was a double room with a wardrobe built into one corner and a standard hospital cupboard in the opposite corner. There was a single bed against the other wall with its head just by the door. The only furniture other than that were four chairs of a mongrel variability and little comfort. There were two windows but each of them was high up against the ceiling with sloping sills. The bright sun that shone all that summer only managed to reach through those windows for a brief time each day. Looking up, all I could see was a small piece of blue sky and part of the upper storey of a nearby building. This room certainly had the feel of a cell rather than a bedroom. However, it seemed somehow appropriate to me. Here I was, in my cell.

That evening one of the night nurses found me a hospital gown but I ignored it. There was no way I was going to wear one of those awful things with the split up the back. Anyway, I felt too apathetic to get changed. I did lie on the bed, at one point pulling the covers over me as it became quite cool in the night. By the time the night nurse did the morning round, looking into each room, I had got up and, one of the chairs being at the end of the bed, I was able to sit sideways and lean across the end of bed, supported on my elbows. The nurse expressed her surprise at my being dressed already. 'Oh, are you up already?' she said, then went away, closing the door behind her.

It must have been some hours later that the door opened. I glanced up briefly, immediately deciding that the person who stood in the doorway was a doctor. I somehow got the impression that he was taking in the rather pathetic scene that met him, though I had looked down again within seconds and continued my previous habit of mindlessly picking fluff off the hospital blanket.

My visitor took a chair, moved it towards me, and sat down, initially saying nothing.

I sat there as I had been doing for some five hours, in a dress I had slept in, hair unbrushed, staring at the bed I had not bothered to make. I had never felt so desolate. I did not want anyone to approach me; I did not want anyone to concern themselves with me. For someone to enter my room, come in and sit down, seemed positively excessive. I wondered why I could not be left alone in that large room at the end. I felt cut off, as it seemed I wanted to be – if only no one would come through the door.

'Hello, Veronica, I'm Nick Rose. I'm the consultant here.'

Oh. I gave a slight nod. Go away, I thought, you are wasting your time, there is no point in anyone coming here. Can you not see how awful it all is? How hopeless?

At that point Karen came in and handed over the medical notes. 'Good morning, Veronica,' she said cheerfully, then left the room. What had she got to be so bloody cheerful about? I thought, why don't they all go away?

'Not the nicest of rooms,' the doctor remarked.

Yes, maybe, but what had niceness to do with all this?

He sat and looked at the notes. That must make interesting reading, I thought; that would indicate how awful I was.

'I've seen you before,' he observed.

I had thought there was something familiar when I had seen him in the doorway, but had not bothered to search my mind for the origins of that feeling. Put to me like that, however, it caused a difficulty – unanswered it prevented resolution of the conversation, such as it was, yet I did not want to make a reply that would encourage further speech. Everything was so confusing to me. I had a sense that it was all unreal.

'I work in High Wycombe,' I replied, not sure if it were relevant.

'Yes,' he said, 'on the special care baby unit. I went there to set up the staff support group.'

Well, I thought, that is ironic. All this just shows how receptive I am to staff support. Now he said it, I remembered him. One of the charge nurses on SCBU had commented on its being a pity that he was moving to Oxford because he was so nice.

He sat there looking at the notes – quiet, calm, unhurried. I noted that there was no attempt to make me explain myself, justify my presence.

'. . . I haven't got any of my things and I don't even know where I am.' I was not even sure that it was I who had said it. Had I said anything else? I did not know. It seemed all so supremely pathetic. The previous evening I had heard someone in the quad comment on the smell of burning stubble. Burning stubble? I had thought, but I was supposed to be in Oxford and they did not burn stubble in cities, did they? It had added to my confusion about where I was, a confusion that I had apparently just expressed. I felt angry with myself for saying something, inviting a response. Why did I not just ignore him so that he would go away?

'Yes, it's very confusing, isn't it.' He leant forwards, towards me, and spoke quietly and calmly.

Where had quietness and calmness come from? I wondered, and how had he managed to say that and sound understanding, not patronising? 'I want to go home,' I said. Here was the real test – would he let me go?

'I don't think you could cope with that right now, do you?'

I had moved slightly towards him, though still looking down; now I moved back again. 'That doesn't matter,' I said.

He had not heard. He leant further forwards in case I should repeat it but I did not. He did not ask me to. He stood up to go and, leaning slightly forwards and speaking quietly again, said, 'I'm Nick Rose. I'm the consultant. Have you got that, Veronica?'

I nodded. I had got that. I also understood that this was someone who recognised how confused I was and had therefore repeated the essential information. Essential? Well, there must have been some point in repeating it, some point in making that effort to break through my confusion.

He paused at the door and said, 'Well, we'll just get to know you over the next few days.' I had glanced up. The door closed; I was alone in my cell again.

Richard came to visit me on the Saturday afternoon. Mike, one of the nurses, showed him to my room. Richard took a chair and moved it away from me before sitting down – the opposite of what

Nick had done, I realised. His first words were harsh. 'I do everything I can to make you happy and this is the result,' he said bitterly and accusingly.

I was distressed by his attitude. When he asked if I wanted him to contact my family I said no, adding that if I could not have him I did not want anyone. At that moment I needed him more than I had ever done before, yet all I got from him were bitter recriminations that I could not cope with. I begged him to forgive me, desperate to have someone familiar to support me, to help me.

Eventually he began to relent and said that he would bring me what I needed from my belongings. I said that I did not want anything. When Richard left he went to find Mike, the nurse in charge, as Mike had asked to see him before he left. Mike invited him to sit down and Richard explained that I was telling him not to bring any of my things and that I did not want anyone in my family informed. This troubled Richard as it made him feel burdened with a situation he might not be able to cope with on his own. As for my belongings, it seemed quite unreasonable not to want anything, always supposing I was going to stay. Mike told him that they were likely to keep me for a while yet so I would need something.

Richard nodded. He found the whole situation very hard to take in. He found it hard to imagine that I was really ill, really needed to be in a psychiatric hospital of all places, after all his mother had been really depressed when she was with us, yet she had recovered in the cottage hospital.

Richard did bring some of my belongings. He also informed my family, first getting in touch with my brother Patrick and sister-in-law Kathleen, as he thought they would understand more. Patrick is a registered nurse of the learning disabled (mentally ill, learning disabled, what's the difference?) and Kath is a social worker.

Once Richard had gone, Mike came to my room. He told me the result of his conversation with Richard, including his assurance that the nursing staff were there for him as well as for me. 'I've been in touch with SCBU and told them that you are in hospital,' he told me.

'I don't want anyone to be told that I am here!' I protested, with a rare look at the person I was talking to.

Mike responded sympathetically but pointed out that it would be unfair to leave them without knowing, as they would have to make arrangements to cover for me. This did not make me feel any better about it.

Over that weekend I was invited by a nurse to come to each meal and to each meeting, or simply to come out and join them. Most of these invitations were ignored, though very occasionally I would venture out and walk up to the quad, walking slowly, head bent down to the floor. I hated cigarettes and the constant odour from staff and patients smoking was highly offensive to me. There wasn't a 'no smoking' area, so I just had to put up with it. The floor was covered with cigarette butts and the chairs were mostly tatty and torn.

Occasionally I was able to go for a walk outside – the occasion, as I came to realise, being when there was a nurse available to accompany me. One nurse who seemed to come to my room more often than any other was a young girl called Andrea. It was Andrea who, several times, was the one who took me for a walk. I remembered her telling me that there used to be a farm in the grounds that the patients used to run. A particular nurse had to come to me quite often before I could identify them. That weekend I also came to recognise Karen, Tim Woodward and Mike. One attribute of Tim and Mike that I found particularly sympathetic was the quietness of their voices. I liked to be spoken to quietly and sympathetically. Nick Rose had spoken to me quietly and sympathetically.

Often when a nurse came to my room, I would be offered a cup of tea. This I would accept but I refused all offers to attend meals and ate nothing whatsoever over the weekend. I did not feel hungry. Over the last few months I had become used to living on practically nothing.

The polite insistence at outpatients that I did not go home, that I did not move my own car and the fact that Stephen had stayed with me at all times, reminded me of that day at school when I was in the sixth form, that I had spent in the bishop's room.

Nevertheless, on the ward I was at first perplexed by the fact that, whenever I left my room and entered the quad, there was invariably a nurse there, even if there was no one else, and that nurse would attach themselves to me, shadowing my every move. No one, as far as I could remember, actually explained close observation to me. Later I found that there were occasions when I was politely told that they did not want me to go beyond a certain point. As I later discovered, this was when they were short-staffed and could not afford one member of staff to absent themselves from the ward to follow me. It was a while before I came to understand the rules of that particular game. It all seemed rather peculiar and added to my sense of unreality. I realised with some confusion that they took me very seriously. They really thought that I might harm myself. But people did not do things like that, did they? But then there was Chris, my brother-in-law Keith's close friend, who had killed himself. He was found dead not long after he had visited Clare and Keith, when he had been laughing and joking. Keith said that his friend had taken the coward's way out, but Clare had disagreed. 'Could you sit in your car and wait for the fumes to kill you?' she had asked. I wondered if I was capable of such a thing. I hoped so – if not, it meant that there was no way out.

On the Sunday I ventured from my room just after everyone had had their breakfast. Someone came up to me and asked if I would like breakfast and I meekly followed them out to the kitchen. There were times when I seemed to run out of the energy to maintain refusals, in which case I would simply do as I was told.

Somehow I found myself alone in the dining room that adjoined the kitchen. I looked around, an achievement in itself since it required me to look up from the floor, and realised that I was indeed alone. Furthermore, I had free access to the area where Stephen had stood with me that first day – and thence to the outside. I was still plagued by thoughts of self-destruction and I knew enough by then to realise that there should have been someone with me. I had a vague feeling that to go away on my own was somehow not to play the game. But then, I thought, I had not been asked to be part of this – who had said I had to be? I had told them before that I wanted to go and they had all ignored me. I wanted no more of this – it was all too awful, and utterly pointless. What was the point of their spending time and energy on me? If only they realised how useless I was, they would not bother with me. They would not bother following me around to save me from myself. Why could they not leave me alone to do what I wanted to do? Well, I thought, it seemed like they had.

I made my way slowly, cautiously, towards the door and walked out into the open. I half-expected someone to arrive, but no one did. Outside it was hot already and the sun was shining brightly. I walked at my usual slow pace, with my eyes to the ground. I went along the edge of the driveway. At one point I felt a bit dizzy, perhaps because of the hot sun, perhaps because of the drugs I was being given. I sat on the kerb for a few minutes and looked around. There was the exit from the hospital, not far away. I heard cars passing at high speed. This was my way out. I got up and made my way, not quickly – I could not have moved quickly if I had tried – but purposely, the sound of the cars attracting me.

When I got to the main gate I was once again taken by an attack of giddiness. There was a low wall there, which I sat on, waiting for the effect to wear off. On the Friday night I had not been given my usual tablets, but another antidepressant, amitriptyline, from which I initially suffered a lot of side effects, dizziness being one of them. I sat on the low wall feeling quite peculiar, waiting for the effects to wear off. I could hear the cars going by fast. As I sat there I was aware of a car coming up the drive, turning quickly, and going back.

I glanced towards the hospital. Jon, the ward manager, and a student nurse were coming towards me. I did not move until they reached me. 'Veronica, can I be an awful bore and ask you to come with us?' Jon said when they reached me.

I went with them; I did not have the energy to protest, much less to run away. I accompanied them back to the ward. What, I wondered, would have happened if I had not done as I was so politely asked? I did not know for sure but I suspected that there would be no advantage in finding out. I was outnumbered. I should have taken the chance when it was offered. I was stupid. I could not even kill myself when the opportunity presented – how was that for failure? So I found myself once more in the quad staring out of the window.

Not long after I had been brought in from the hospital gates, someone came to me and told me that I had a visitor. I turned around. It was Hugh. He smiled and said hello. We went to my room and talked generally for a while, with me speaking quietly and slowly as ever.

Before he went, he picked up my Bible. Richard had, following his conversation with Mike, brought in some clothes and other things for me. He had known me well enough to be aware that I would want my Bible and had taken it from where it always sat, next to my bed. Hugh read the story of Mary weeping by Jesus' tomb. Mary was weeping because 'They have taken away my Lord and I do not know where they have put him.' To me, it was a very familiar story. My father had often told it to me when I was a child. Hugh said that Mary was crying because she had lost something, something very precious and I, it seemed, had also lost something precious.

Hugh left, saying that he was just about to go away on holiday. I thought that it was good of him to come to visit me and I felt comforted by his presence, and by what he said.

I soon discovered that the blue room was a place where I would be allowed to stay on my own for a short while. Inevitably, however, someone would come and check on me. While I was alone there one day, I noticed that the windows were long sash ones that reached almost to the floor. It occurred to me that if I opened the window I could just step out. I pushed the window up; it went a short way then stopped. Looking up, I realised that wooden pieces had been screwed into place so that the window only opened so far – and not far enough to allow for climbing out. 'Damn!' I thought, 'they think of everything in this place.'

One day I went through to the blue room and sat, head in hands, feeling utterly desolate. Someone came through and sat back on his heels in front of me. I raised my eyes just far enough to see that it was Mike. 'I feel like crying, but I can't,' I said.

'It'll come,' he said, quietly and sympathetically.

During the first week I received a beautiful bouquet of flowers from my brothers and sisters, and an arrangement from my mother. Throughout the two months of that first admission, I had at least two vases of flowers in my room. I kept receiving flowers, arrangements, plants, cards and letters. I arranged the flowers and cards around the large room on the floor as there was nowhere else for them to go. The cleaning lady said that she did not like going into my room in case she disturbed them, and also, the room was so tidy. Never in subsequent admissions did I ever receive so much. Was it that never again people would feel such sympathy?

Chapter 7

Interview with registrar who suggests ECT – Nick Rose
intervenes – Groups – Second interview with registrar – ECT
– Nick Rose intervenes again

Every day in Phoenix started with a community meeting which
everyone was expected to attend, staff and patients alike. It lasted
for an hour from 10.00, at least theoretically; in fact, the ward
round, which took place in the blue room on Mondays and Fridays,
usually went on beyond 10.00. That Monday morning the patients
who were waiting in the quad complained to the nursing staff that
the community meeting was having to begin late once again because
of the ward meeting. The nursing staff sympathised but said there
was not much that they could do about it. Eventually the ward
round finished and they were able to enter the blue room for the
community meeting.

I was in my room having, as usual, ignored the invitation to the
community meeting. Later, however, there was a knock on the door
and a woman I did not recognise entered. 'Veronica,' she asked,
'would you like to come with me and meet Dr Courtenay?'

I entered the room slowly, with head bowed, my slowness of

movement and thought – psychomotor retardation – itself being indicative of the depth of my depression. I sat down as requested, wringing my hands and curled up as usual, with my face hidden.

'Hello, Veronica,' the registrar said. 'We have been talking about you in the ward round. We are very concerned about you. The nurses who have been looking after you this weekend are very worried. It is clear that you are seriously depressed. Do you know what that means?'

I nodded and said, in a whisper that made Nigel Courtenay lean forward to hear, 'I have had it before.'

'Yes, I know. I telephoned Salisbury but did not find out much other than that it seems to have lasted quite a long time. I notice that you are speaking very quietly – you are difficult to hear – the nurses say that it is rare for you to speak at all. You rarely come out of your room and have eaten nothing since you have been here. All this points to your being very depressed. You could help yourself, though, by spending time outside your room, talking to the nurses and eating properly.'

Throughout this, I remained silent and unresponsive.

'Now, it is imperative that we start effective treatment as soon as possible. You have already started antidepressants, which is good, but they take too long to be effective and your state is such that you need a treatment that is immediate as well as efficient. That treatment is ECT.'

It was with profound shock that I heard him introduce the subject of electro-convulsive therapy. ECT? I could find no words to express myself, but I began to shake my head in refusal and disbelief.

'Why are you refusing?' the doctor asked.

I simply persisted in shaking my head. I did not want it; I would not have it. He continued, persistently, persuasively. 'The nursing staff can see someone who is obviously in great distress. ECT is very effective; its effect is immediate, unlike drugs that take time to work. The nurses do not like to see someone in so much distress. You stay in your room all on your own most of the time, and will not speak to anyone. You are not eating, at least you are drinking, but you are obviously very distressed and need a treatment that is immediately effective. We are really concerned about you and we want to relieve the distress that is all too obvious. Do you know what ECT is?'

I nodded. I felt angry, angry and betrayed. It seemed that the nurses had been watching and noting my behaviour since I had arrived, telling everything to this doctor to pressurise me, for I felt pressurised. They had not told me that they were watching me.

'Have you seen it?'

I nodded once more. Like many nurses, I had seen the procedure during the psychiatric secondment of my general training.

'What are your objections?'

'I don't want it!' I said, my voice full of emotion. I was alarmed. I felt threatened, pressurised. I did not want it – was that not enough? No, it was not, for the doctor continued.

'Veronica, I really do not think that you are in your right mind. I do not think that you are in a fit state to judge this issue.'

An answer for everything, I thought.

'I really think you ought to trust us,' Dr Courtenay added.

Trust them? I thought. But no one will listen to me! No one will speak for me. The senior house officer just sat there, as did the nurse, apparently going along with everything that Dr Courtenay said. I could look for no support from there. And Dr Courtenay was so persuasive, so very persistent. I felt besieged and was aware of not representing myself very well. But how could I? I was scared of ECT, scared of having an anaesthetic, scared of being so much at the mercy of others, scared of people who would not listen – did not think it necessary to listen. This was madness, if you could not think straight, could not explain yourself. It meant that you could be ignored, your views bypassed. Your opinion might be sought out of courtesy but it was really just a charade and could be set aside, ignored. No one would stand up for me, no one would represent me. I was frightened, but could not explain myself. I just knew that I did not want ECT, but the doctor would not give in – insistent, persuasive – I felt pressurised. I was scared, confused. Was I mad? I thought I must be, otherwise I would have said something sensible, explained myself, defended myself.

'You went to the main gates on Sunday,' Dr Courtenay commented, 'were you going towards the road?'

What? I thought, going for the road? Who had said I was? How did he know? Was he anything to do with the car that had backed up? He seemed to know what had been going through my mind. How did he know that? He was right, of course, and he obviously took it seriously, he obviously understood. Yet ECT? How could no one understand about ECT?

'Now, this isn't a threat,' Dr Courtenay said carefully, leaning towards me, gesturing with his hand, 'but you know we can treat you without your consent'.

I felt quite simply scared. It seemed that my refusal was an inconvenience that could be argued aside, whatever the objection. If all else failed, if I maintained my inconvenient attitude it could be ignored altogether. Not a threat? I had never felt so threatened in all my life – anxiety was rapidly being replaced by a sense of panic. It did not matter what I thought. No one would support my view because it was irrelevant. Any semblance of respect for my autonomy, my ability to express my views, my feelings, was about to be dispensed with because it had become inconvenient. It seemed to me that I had for months been desperately fighting to retain some semblance of control over my actions, control over my environment – but now I was going to be deprived of any vestige of control that remained. They did not understand. There was only one thing I could do. I actually looked up at Dr Courtenay. 'Could I see Dr Rose?' I asked.

'Yes,' he answered, 'certainly you can see Dr Rose.'

Well, that much had been conceded.

'We will get him to see you as soon as possible,' he added.

Why the rush? I thought, then remembered that I had been told that ECT was given on Tuesdays and Fridays. That day was Monday. Yes, I could see Nick but that was not to be allowed to interfere with their plans. I knew that I could ask to see the consultant – but what if he took the same line? They wanted me to see him before the next day because the next day was Tuesday and on Tuesday I was going to have ECT whether I liked it or not.

My request had at least given me a reprieve – it had stopped Dr Courtenay from being insistent. But would it stop them giving me ECT without my consent? I would not sign a consent form; I would not let them anaesthetise me. The idea that the Mental Health Act should be used on me seemed quite unreal – only people who were seriously ill needed that.

I waited all day to see Nick Rose. I waited for someone to be calm and quiet, to listen to me, to hear me and respond to what I said. I hardly knew why I was so confident about it, so prepared to wait; one thing was certain, though, the acute anxiety that had built up into alarm lessened as I waited. For some reason it did not occur to me to worry that Nick might take the same approach as his registrar.

Mike was the nurse with me that day. I found him easy to recognise with a glance, for he had dark hair and such blue eyes and he always spoke quietly to me. I preferred people to speak quietly to me; quietness was calmness, it gave me confidence. I hated loud noises of any nature.

I was told that Nick was not in Oxford that afternoon, but they would get him to see me as soon as he returned. I felt as if I was playing a part in some elaborate charade. Why had the registrar bothered to speak to me that morning? Talk about consent? Why did he not simply say 'we have decided to give you ECT tomorrow, we do not care whether you sign a consent form or not'? Why did he not say 'your opinion does not matter because we have decided what to do and if you do not like it, we will section you'?

Why not simply say that and have done with it?

That afternoon the registrar asked the nursing staff to bleep him when Nick arrived, so it was that he accompanied the consultant when he went to see me. Nick greeted me with a reassuring smile. I, the two doctors and Mike, my nurse, went through to the blue room.

I began to speak, in fact I spoke so much that I amazed myself. To me, this was my last chance. It was my only chance, and I was going to make the best of it. I said that if I did whatever was asked of me, agreed with what was said to me, then I was displaying insight, was in my right mind. If I disagreed, however, then I was not in my right mind, could not make decisions for myself, was not in a fit state. When I said that I did not want ECT, I was told that my opinion did not matter anyway, they could go ahead without my agreement.

Nick, leaning towards me and listening carefully, noting the anxiety, desperation even, in my voice, interrupted me. 'We will not do anything that you do not agree to,' he told me.

I was amazed. I had never been so relieved to hear something said in all my life. He was saying that they would have to consult me, really consult me, listen to what I said, respect my view. Here was someone who was prepared to see me, to listen to me, to respect what I said – and he said that they would not force me.

I went on, defending myself, explaining myself, trying to show that I was not just being unreasonable (mad?). I told Nick how confused I was, though I thought he knew that, had seen it from the start when he had visited me that first morning. I pointed out that I had never seen that hospital before. It was unfamiliar, the people were unfamiliar – he was the only person in that place whom I had ever seen before. They wanted me to speak to the nurses, but I felt . . . Here I paused, unable to say what I wanted to say.

Nick was about to say something but Nigel put up his hand and, sensing that this was something important, prompted me. 'Felt? Felt what?'

'I feel . . . I feel as if there are two groups of people – inadequate people who can't cope and successful nurses doing their jobs.' *I, of course, was in the former category.* Well, I had said it and was glad that I had. It sounded crazy but it was true. I was grateful to have been encouraged to say it; it had been weighing on my mind. Now I had said it, perhaps someone could help me to get past that awful barrier. I was surprised that it was Nigel Courtenay who had intervened to get that out – as if he knew how important it was. Did he do it because he thought that there was something important there? Did he do it because he thought it would be helpful? Or because he was curious, interested? It did not really matter.

He had allowed me to say it and I felt relieved that I had done so.

Nick Rose went on to explain about ECT and drugs. They were usually equally effective but ECT gave much quicker results. He admitted that he thought I ought to have ECT, that it was the right treatment.

'But,' I responded, 'I am taking all the drugs I've been prescribed – even the chlorpromazine, though I don't really like taking that.'

'Well,' he answered, 'you needn't take it. It was only prescribed to help you sleep.'

Now come on, I thought, don't start giving me choices where I do not really want them – I only brought that up to show how good I am being. I certainly did not want to go back to lying awake for hours. The chlorpromazine guaranteed, for the first time in months, that when I went to bed I would go to sleep.

While they were on the subject of drugs, I pointed out that my drug prescription had been changed without my knowledge or consent. I added that I had taken the drugs despite no one's thinking it necessary to inform me of what was happening.

Nick looked around at his colleagues and suggested, 'We need to improve our communications.'

I took this as a welcome sign that I was at least speaking sense. 'I'm feeling all light-headed and I keep getting palpitations,' I said.

Nick explained that they would be increasing the dose quite quickly, but it was necessary and that it would help if I could put up with the side-effects. I was being given the full dose in one at night so that the worst of the side-effects would be over by the morning.

This, I thought, was news to me. So far all anyone had spoken about was ECT. At this point Dr Courtenay interposed, saying that they had earlier discussed other things that I could do to help myself. That was true, I thought, and maybe it contradicts what I just thought about ECT.

Nick agreed that that was important.

'I don't like sitting with everyone else. They all smoke.' I defended myself, though rather disingenuously – smoke did not prevent me from sitting with the others when I wanted their company, later in my admission. 'I know I don't sit and watch television with the others but I never watch it, even at home.' This was true; the television invariably stayed off until Richard came in and switched it on.

The subject of my spending most of my time in my room was brought up, and the fact that I was not eating. And what about the groups? I should go to them. Nick once more agreed with this.

Before they finished their discussion, however, Nick warned me that ECT might have to be reconsidered. 'I know it does not seem as if it could get worse, but if, for example, you were to stop drinking . . .' he explained. It did not alarm me so much then, for he had promised me that they would not do anything without my consent. I noticed the comment that it may not seem to me as if it could get worse – it was something else that suggested he understood how things felt for me.

So the interview ended. I had a sense of having been listened to, I had been able to say what I wanted to say, express what I needed to express. I had been allowed to communicate my difficulties. I did not want ECT. I wanted time, that is what I needed, *time*. Time to adjust, time to work through that awful confusion, time to work out my feelings, my guilt, my *shame* at being there. I was a nurse, not a patient – wasn't I? No, I could not be, I could not be a nurse. I had made such a mess of it all. I was a patient, a patient in a psychiatric hospital. Was I mad? Surely you would have to be mad to think like I did. This was a psychiatric hospital – that was where they put mad people, wasn't it? They would not let me go, I knew that for certain. Even Dr Rose would not stand aside and let me walk out of there. But he had listened to me. He had understood that I was not just being awkward. He had told me the truth. He thought that I should have ECT, but he had given me the choice, the choice to do things my way. Could I do it my way?

Richard had not been involved in any of this so far, but Dr Courtenay came to my room on the Wednesday to ask me if the telephone number he had for Richard was correct as he could not get through. 'I don't want Richard to know about this,' I said. I did not want anyone to know about anything – just go away.

'I think you ought to let me be the judge of that,' he replied.

Here we are again, I thought, being told I am not in a fit state of mind to make decisions for myself. When Richard did come, he said, 'Can't they do anything other than drug you out of your mind or electrify your brain? It's barbaric!' It was not a helpful comment in itself, but it reflected his concern.

I tried to go to meals, to spend more time out of my room, to go to the groups – but it was all so hard. They wanted me to behave as if I was part of it all but I did not feel as if I were. I ate meals as I had been told to, because I had been told to, but I did not feel hungry and found it impossible to feel as if there were any point in taking nourishment. I went out into the quadrangle but continued to sit on the table in the corner, keeping away from the other patients. Sometimes I sat in the circle of people – nurses, patients, sometimes doctors – who were usually there, but I found it so difficult. It made me feel exposed, vulnerable. I sat on the edge of the seat, curled up, looking down, wringing my hands, hoping that no one would say anything to me. But they did, they kept doing it – could they not see that I wanted to be left alone? Could they not see what a waste of time it all was? When someone did speak to me, I tried to summon up the courage and energy to reply. Sometimes I would simply nod, or shake my head – then turn myself away, hoping that they would give up and go away. If I said anything in reply, it was rarely more than a whispered word or two.

I liked most to be in my room, sat on the bed, swinging my legs. Richard was going to bring my radio, some books and my Scrabble. I usually loved reading, listening to the radio, but I found it so difficult then. I could not concentrate, could not think straight. The most simple things confused and confounded me. Sometimes I would just sit and rock myself gently, like a baby, finding comfort in the simple motion.

At least my sleeping was better with the chlorpromazine. All I needed do was to wait, wait to become drowsy, then fall to sleep.

When I was out of my room, I would sometimes lean on the high windowsill at the end of the corridor and look out of the window. Or I would stand looking out at the courtyard through the window in the quad. I liked to look outside; that was where I wanted to be. I felt penned in and wanted to be outside. If there was a nurse free they would go for a walk around the grounds with me. The grounds were beautiful and extensive. One day I was out for a walk with Mike when I heard a train going by in the near distance. I remarked that psychiatric hospitals often seemed to be built near railway lines. Mike said that it was probably something to do with such hospitals often being built near the edge of towns.

I sat down on the grass and Mike did also. I talked about the depressed man whom I had met as a student nurse and how I had spoken to him to give him hope. I wondered aloud whether I had done the right thing and Mike expressed the view that the man had been suffering from a treatable illness, in which case I had done the right thing to give him support, to help him benefit from that treatment. Well, maybe, I thought, perhaps that was one way of looking at it.

Mike said that we ought to go back, and got up to go. I did not. I sat, looking at the ground. I did not want to go. I did not want to go when Mike wanted me to go. Why? I did not know. A protest, perhaps. Why did I have to go the moment someone else decided I should go?

Mike asked me to come. I shook my head. There was a pause. Mike was giving me a bit of time to think about it, I thought. I did not move. 'Come on, Veronica,' he said, in a quite different tone. Enough was enough, he was being serious. We were going. I got up. We returned to the ward.

Would I have felt better if Mike had accepted my 'I will stay here as long as I like' and waited? I thought not. Actually I would probably have been somewhat alarmed. I needed boundaries and I wanted to know where they were. If Mike had responded with uncertainty, not knowing whether or when to assert some control over the situation, it would have been the most disastrous of all. I needed to know where the boundaries were, and to feel safe.

There was also, of course, the fact that I had chosen to make my small rebellion while in Mike's care. I was beginning to know the nurses and was able to identify the experienced ones, those with whom I could feel the most safe.

Why then did a section for ECT not make me feel safe? Why was it not better to have someone making that decision, marking that particular boundary on my behalf, making me feel safe? It was not because the former was more trivial, for even the smallest things presented great problems – problems to be made sense of, sorted out, understood.

The advantage with ECT was supposed to be that it was quickly effective. Yet, if I could not cope with how I felt that day, how could I cope with feeling quite different tomorrow? In addition, taking away my right to determination seemed to me highly alarming; particularly when I had not yet decided whether I was safe outside the door. Perhaps the final truth was that, at that moment, anaesthetics, ECT and sections quite simply frightened me. I felt scared, threatened.

Nick Rose had said that he thought I should have ECT. But he had not insisted. He did not insist because of what I thought, felt. He had not ruled it out entirely, though. He had told me that if I got worse, they would have to reconsider the question. 'I know it does not seem as if you could get worse,' he had said, in sympathetic recognition of how awful I felt – he was not making a threat of what might happen – 'but if, for instance, you stopped drinking . . .' Yes, I knew that would be serious, that made sense. Then, he had said, they would have to consider ECT again.

So, there it was. He had promised that nothing would be done against my will. I had said that I did not want ECT. He had said that I would have to have it if things got worse. How did that add up? If I was determined to resist ECT at all costs, how could he keep his promise that nothing would be done without my consent? Simple, of course. He would persuade me to sign a consent form. Could he do that? Yes, I rather thought he could. I was not entirely comfortable with that idea.

Thinking of this I remembered what Dr Rose had said at the end of our interview in the blue room.

'Do you think you *deserve* to get well?' he had asked, stressing the '*deserve*'.

Deserve to get well? What had that got to do with anything? There was no such thing as 'deserve' in my life, it was an irrelevance. I shrugged my shoulders slightly and shook my head in reply, as much in confusion as in denial.

'I do, I think you *deserve* to get well.' A clear, simple statement. He would not say anything unless it were true, would he? No, I thought, he would not. So how was I to make sense of that one? I had not understood it then. I understood it better when I thought of it, but I did not know how to believe it. However, it showed great understanding of the beliefs that dominated my thoughts.

I told Richard what Nick had said and he thought it very odd. Jenni, SCBU's bereavement counsellor, understood straight away and responded, 'What a lovely thing to say!' She understood the extreme guilt and sense of undeservedness that went with depression. It was part of our tragedy that Richard was struggling for any sort of understanding.

I went away from the interview feeling that I had escaped, but only just. I worried about the question of whether I might get worse. I had asked for time and space to see if I could improve things. I had been given it and would have to put everything I had into using it.

I started to attend meetings, though not without a supreme effort. There was a community meeting, 10.00–10.45 weekdays and 10.00–10.30 weekends. I hated community meetings – too many people, too long, too much of a challenge. Then, of course, there was the ward diary, the previous day's entry, written by staff or patients, was read out at the beginning of the meeting. During the first few weeks I found that I was mentioned in it almost every day – 'Veronica is still very low' – 'Veronica is spending a lot of time in her room' – 'Veronica is still very quiet' etc. etc. I could cheerfully (ambitious as that may have been) have put a match to it.

It took all the courage I could muster to walk into the room. I felt so afraid. I sat, hunched up, looking at the floor, unable to look up, unable to face anyone, praying that no one would speak to me, would notice me – and then they would read that wretched diary. How could I escape notice when they deliberately drew attention to me? It seemed cruel to me. How was it supposed to help me, putting me through that ordeal day after day? I could not believe that forcing me to push myself into an experience that made me feel so awful could be in any way beneficial. I kept going to the community meetings but it never seemed to get easier.

Initially I failed to respond at all if someone spoke to me. Gradually I found the courage to respond, but things seemed to improve so gradually. At first, I would simply nod or shake my head. I then began to answer verbally, albeit quietly and while maintaining my stare at the floor. I still needed to push myself though, and push myself hard.

The women's group and the small group were a bit easier in that there were fewer people to face when I entered the room. But of course, that also meant there were fewer people to detract attention from me. Eventually it was the small group, on Tuesdays, that proved most helpful, but it was a long time before I became aware of that.

Twelve days after ECT had been proposed, I attended the women's group. I found the group difficult and became very tense and anxious. I was unable to respond when addressed and it was all I could do to stop from running out. When it finally came to an end, I stayed in the blue room while the others went through to the quad. Realising that I was missing, one of the nurses came to find me. She tried to persuade me to go through and join everyone in the quad, but I obdurately refused. I covered my face with my hands and refused even to look up. The nurse asked me if I would like a cup of tea, but I shook my head. I simply wanted to be left alone. The nurse tried once more to persuade me to go through but I once more refused.

The nurse went away but was soon replaced by Emma, the nurse in charge that day. I was confused by her presence. I could not think clearly enough to realise that there was a connection between her immediate appearance following on from the other nurse's exit. Emma knelt beside me and tried to persuade me to go through to the quad and offered me a cup of tea, but to neither suggestion did I respond, in any way.

Suddenly Emma got up, saying, 'I'm going to get Nigel.' At that moment it did not register with me what she had actually said. Emma was replaced by the other nurse, who simply stayed with me.

I was dismayed when Nigel Courtenay arrived – what was he doing here? He pulled a chair up in front of me and sat down, leaning towards me sat there, curled up and staring at the carpet. He started to ask questions. I felt decidedly suspicious – what was going on?

When Dr Courtenay put it to me that I was much worse that day I began to feel frightened and vulnerable. Once again I felt the lack of someone there to speak for me, to be with me. I felt angry with the nurse for just sitting there. So much for the patient advocate. I felt exposed and isolated.

Dr Courtenay commented on the fact that I was not looking at him at all, where previously I had at least looked up occasionally.

Commenting on my refusal of the invitation to have a cup of tea he said that I was not even drinking. When I answered 'it doesn't matter' to something that Nigel said, he suggested that it was a sign of deterioration, since I had not said that previously. 'You know we can section you and give you treatment without your consent – wouldn't it be so much nicer if you signed a consent form?'

'Well, I will get Dr Rose for you,' Dr Courtenay said after a pause. I noted that he was willing to concede that without my asking. Why not? Like asking my opinion of ECT, it did not really matter. It was a formality that need not get in the way.

Dr Courtenay left. Emma had disappeared from the scene by then, though the original nurse was there. Someone else arrived. He knelt down by me as Emma had done. He explained that we had not met before, and introduced himself as Martin. It seemed incredible to me that there could be anyone on the ward whom I had not met.

Martin once more tried to persuade me to go through to the quad and have a cup of tea. This time I responded, for no more positive a reason than that I might as well for I felt defeated, beaten. I was afraid and there was no one who cared – so long as I did what I was told and had ECT. They told me that they were there to help me, to look after me, to help me recover from my illness. (It was they who said that I was ill, not me.) Yet here I was again, isolated, with no one to speak for me, to defend me.

It was not until later that afternoon that Nick Rose arrived with Dr Courtenay. I had obediently stayed in the quad, although I sat on the table in the corner, away from all the others. I supposed that Nick had come to see me but he did not approach me. Instead he joined the circle of patients and nurses. He took part in the conversation, then turned to where I sat and said, 'Come and join us.' He pulled a chair up on his left and invited me to sit there.

I felt nervous and self-conscious. I had expected Nick to stand up and ask me to go through to the blue room but he kept talking and listening, quite casually. There was a pot of tea on the table and someone offered me a cup. I accepted with a nod – I dare not refuse, given the events earlier in the day.

The trolley arrived for tea and people started to drift through to the kitchen. At least three different people invited me to come to tea. I shook my head each time. I felt as if I could scream – did they not realise that Nick had come to see me? The last thing I wanted was a postponement. I wanted to know the worst.

When everyone had gone but Nick Rose, Dr Courtenay and me, Nick turned to me. 'I'm told that you're much worse today. Is that true?' A question, I noted, not a statement.

I played with the empty cup in my hand. I then actually glanced up and met his eyes for just a brief moment before returning to stare at the floor. 'I'm just having a bad day – sometimes I do. It's no worse than days I've had before. It's just a bad day, that's all.' As usual he needed to lean forwards to hear me, though I had at least managed to look up at him. Not looking up had been one of the things held against me that morning.

'Hmmm,' Nick said, thoughtfully. Getting to his feet he said, 'Well, we'll see tomorrow.' With that he left the room followed by Dr Courtenay. Another reprieve.

I must have been 'better' the next day as no doctors came to talk to me about ECT. It puzzled me that apparently no one came to assess the situation, though as a nurse it should have occurred to me that my behaviour was being noted and discussed among all members of the team. I was still perplexed by my inability to understand what would otherwise have been obvious.

It was the last I heard from the medical staff concerning ECT.

Chapter 8

Nurses try to persuade me to have ECT – Tim intervenes –
Mother's first visit – Richard's visit – I leave unit for two
hours – Rob calls the police

When I walked slowly out of my room one morning, in my familiar
stance with eyes fixed to the ground, it was to find Martin sitting
in the quad. By this time I had worked out the significance of the
one person sat there waiting for my appearance. Martin followed
me to the kitchen. 'It's really good to see you eating,' he remarked
as I helped myself to cereal. I nodded in acknowledgement of his
comment.

After eating my cereal I walked into the big room between the
medical office and the quad. It was large but almost empty, the
only furniture being a television fixed to the wall in one corner and
a few chairs. No one seemed to watch the television though it was
sometimes on. The room seemed to be used as little more than a
corridor from the medical office to the rest of the ward. I went to
one of the windows, leaned on the sill and looked out. The sun was
once again beating down and it was hot already.

'Would you like to go out?' Martin asked.

I nodded. We went out of the door in the low security corridor, open as usual, and into the walled courtyard with its immense horse chestnut trees. 'We'll stay in the courtyard,' Martin said. Having been away for two days he preferred to get the feel of my mood before he was too adventurous. 'Why don't you want ECT?' he asked, as we walked alongside each other.

I simply shook my head, irritated. He continued on the subject of ECT, earnestly trying to convince me that I should consent to it. Eventually I no longer tried to explain myself and just kept quiet. I sat down on the ground, head in hands. After a brief time I stood up and walked towards the door. Martin followed me as I went indoors and across the quad. He stood at the end of the corridor as I walked down to my room, went in and closed the door.

When I did not reappear for some time, Martin came to check on me and to offer me a drink. I was sitting on the edge of the high bed looking at my feet as I swung them back and forth. I accepted the offer of a cup of tea with a nod. He took the cup down to my room and placed it carefully on the chair by the bed, to receive a barely heard thank you.

The nurses supported ECT. So strongly did they believe in it that they felt they should persuade me to agree to it. There was one exception to this. After the first discussion with Nick Rose concerning ECT, Mike, who was my nurse that day, explained about ECT and what would happen if I agreed to have it. I was impressed that Mike took the trouble to explain the procedure in a manner that suggested I was a sane person who could consider and respond rationally, in some degree at least, and not a crazy person who could not think straight or see things sensibly.

He then asked, 'If I say "ECT" what is your gut reaction?'

'No!' I answered emphatically.

'Fair enough,' Mike answered. He raised the subject with me no more. Because of this, he soon became my favourite nurse to be with. Tim, likewise, respected my feelings and did not push the issue.

I found I was having a difficult time with the other nurses. They all seemed to see specialling (being allocated specifically to my care) me as a chance to pressurise me on the subject of ECT. I felt coerced and threatened, and the situation began to cause me real distress. I suspected that they hoped that if they put sufficient pressure on me, they could force me into accepting ECT. It seemed to me that they simply were not receptive to a contrary view. If they are so keen on it, I thought, why don't they volunteer for it? Of course, it was easy for them to recommend it – I would have it as long as they were in the queue before me.

I liked to go outside into the open air; there were times when being inside felt claustrophobic. When I could actually go outside depended on how well staffed the ward was when I made my request. There were days when I was restricted to the quad because they could not allocate a nurse to me alone. On days like this I would often pace up and down the quad. At the time there was another patient in Phoenix who was under close observation and she also employed this means of containing her frustration, so there would be two of us walking to and fro. It was inevitably a source of irritation for some of the other patients, some of whom would leave the quad as a result. Sometimes, however, it worked the other way round; once a patient decided to get rid of her tension by screaming loudly. I, always sensitive to loud sounds, retreated to my room. Not long afterwards, a nurse came down to tell me that they had asked the patient to go into the blue room so it was now all right for me to return to the quad. Despite this, I chose to stay in my room.

I particularly valued those times when there were sufficient staff for me to be accompanied on a walk around the grounds. The grounds included cricket and football pitches, large lawns, courtyards and mature trees. One day I was out in the courtyard with a nurse either side. Each of them decided that this was an opportunity to persuade me to accept ECT. Of course, they knew best, I thought with resentful irony. I was just a patient with the audacity to contradict the people who knew better than me. I really needed to go out whenever I could, yet now it seemed that even my walks were to be used to pressurise me. I put my hands up to my ears unable to endure any further demands. 'Don't talk about ECT!' I pleaded with anguish, my voice almost reaching normal levels.

The nurses, startled by the distress I displayed, went quiet.

From the very first time the possibility had been raised, I had felt pressurised and vulnerable. I had been able to express to Nick my sense of feeling coerced in the face of insistent pressure. At that point, it had come from the medical staff. Now it seemed that the nurses had combined to assert further pressure. It increased my sense of isolation and insecurity. It seemed to me that the nurses were only interested in one thing. I thought, they tell me that I am not in a fit state to make my own decisions, yet they put me in a position where I feel unsafe, then tell me that everything is being done in my best interests. I felt frightened, but also angry and resentful. It appeared that even my infrequent walks were to be exploited, so ruining any relief I gained from them.

There tended to be many fewer patients on the ward at a weekend, as some went home on leave. Tim was on one weekend when it was particularly quiet so he decided that they would have the community meeting in the quad rather than the blue room. I was there, curled up on myself as usual. I found the whole experience frightening and it took a great effort of will for me to be there. Apart from the fact that it took a supreme effort, taking part in the meeting by speaking would draw attention to me when my whole physical stance made me as small and unnoticeable as possible: For although I was attending the meetings, I had never said anything in any of them.

On that particular day, given that the community meeting was much smaller than usual and was being held in the more informal atmosphere of the quad, Tim decided to see if he could induce me to take part in some degree at least. Tim was not one of those nurses who had tried to press me into accepting ECT. I found his quietly spoken manner reassuring. He addressed me, on what subject I cannot remember, but it required an answer. I made a supreme effort to answer and to be heard. He put some more questions to me. I did speak, albeit with my eyes downcast as usual, with only the briefest glances upwards, and in a very quiet voice. It was absurd, really, how difficult I found it to speak with all those people around. (How many people? I don't know, but two would have seemed too many to me.) It was ridiculous how much courage it took for me to answer those questions – how pathetic, how feeble, how scared.

Once the meeting ended, Tim came over to where I was sat. He sat back on his heels to speak to me, curled up as I was. 'Well done, that must have been very difficult,' he said sympathetically.

Absurd and irrational as my difficulties in speaking had seemed to me, Tim seemed to be aware of them. Well done? Had I really done well? He had said I had, he seemed to appreciate my difficulties. Here was another person, as well as Mike, treating me as if I had some rationality somewhere. Those who felt it necessary to put pressure on me to make me agree to ECT made me feel frightened and threatened. Their apparent efforts to make me see sense confirmed the view I had of myself as illogical, awkward and irrational, someone whose only hope was to abandon self-determination. Tim, though, had approached me as if I had achieved something, done something sensible. Much later he told me that he had set up the situation deliberately in order to see if he could induce me to speak.

It was because of Tim's sympathetic approach that I felt able to talk to him regarding the pressure put on me to accept ECT. 'They keep trying to persuade me all the time. It's not fair. I've spoken to the doctors, Dr Rose said I needn't have it and he's the consultant. Even the nursing assistants do it.'

'Well, the nursing assistants are as much a part of the team as everyone else,' Tim commented. I was mildly irritated by this lesson in equality that seemed to have little to do with the point I was making. I found it difficult to believe that the experienced and qualified staff did not know more about ECT than the nursing assistants – or did they not cover ECT in the psychiatric curriculum?

'Some nurses don't agree with ECT,' I pointed out.

Tim nodded. He looked at me. In my whole stance and in everything I said he got the impression, he told me later, of someone who was very afraid. 'I'll speak to the nurses,' he promised. 'Can I suggest you write a statement about this in the diary to be read at the community meeting tomorrow?' Noticing the frown on my face he said, 'I'll leave that up to you.'

I did not feel that I could write in the diary, and thereby possibly induce another discussion on the matter. If I never heard of ECT again, it would be too soon. I was relieved to leave it in Tim's hands. At last I could be with a nurse and they would not bring up the awful subject. I was aware that I was lucky that of the two persons who had sympathy with me in this matter were the consultant and a charge nurse.

What if the pressure had been maintained? I thought, would I have given in and had ECT? After all, my signing a consent form would have made it much nicer for everyone, as Nigel Courtenay had pointed out. Nicer, no doubt, but how important was niceness and quickness?

The controversy had made me lose trust in some of the nursing staff and it took some time for that trust to be restored, which was unfortunate. It was a pity that ECT dominated those first few days on Phoenix. There were so many things that seemed to threaten me and added to my confusion. One of those things was the nurse/patient dichotomy. I was with Tim one day when a woman who was an outpatient asked if I were a patient or a nurse. The patient assumed the two to be mutually exclusive. Since I was undoubtedly a patient there was only one conclusion to be reached. As I became more communicative and patients began to speak to me, I hoped ardently that no one would ask me what my job was. A nurse? Me? What a joke. It was something I became supremely sensitive about.

Clare and Keith, living on Arborfield Garrison near Reading, were very good at coming to visit although it was quite a distance to Littlemore. My cousin Jenny regularly visited from Thame. One day she arrived with her daughter Helen and her niece, my cousin Peter's daughter, Lisa. Melanie came to my room to tell me that they were there, to find me distressed and crying as if I would never stop. Seeing the state I was in, she took my visitors away to sit in the quad while I tried to make myself look decent. However, when I did present myself I must still have looked dreadful, with red, puffy eyes.

Later that day I asked Melanie if I could see Emma, the nurse in charge. I had decided that I was going home. I cannot remember exactly what had happened to bring this on, though I know I was angry for some reason. Melanie passed the message on to Emma, who came to my room. At that time I still felt suspicious of Emma, because of her action in getting Nigel Courtenay to decide that I was worse and needed ECT. I was angry, I was going to go home and no one was going to stop me, least of all Emma. I was quite determined that I was not going to be taken in, to allow Emma to deflect me from my purpose.

Although I was not aware of it at the time, Emma was tremendously helpful and patient. Feeling as I did then, I do not know what I would have done without her. I remember being very agitated and pacing around the room as Emma sat on the bed and spoke to me. At one point I got out my photograph album and opened it at a picture of Clare, Keith and Chris, his friend. I sat and looked at it, not saying anything. Eventually Emma asked who they were. I told her, then started to talk about Chris and how he had killed himself.

We were interrupted by someone who said that I had visitors. Emma suggested that I go and splash water on my face, which looked even worse than it had earlier. My visitors were Keith and Clare.

Emma had persuaded me against going home that evening, saying that she did not think that the doctors would be happy about my leaving. She would talk to them the next morning, so could I wait until then? The next day no one came to talk to me about going home – they seemed to have forgotten all about it. It all seemed rather strange. I was puzzled. Without the desperation of extreme mental distress, I did not have the courage to insist. I stayed.

In retrospect I think it might have been that day that resulted in my mother's first eventful visit. I suspect that Jenny and Clare each telephoned her on the same day, concerned about how they found me in the hospital. Mother had not visited me earlier, as she and various other members of my family had been on a long-planned holiday in Cornwall. She had been trying to persuade me to join them for some months prior to my admission. I had resisted; the last thing I could cope with was a merry family holiday. Apart from Clare, Keith and Jenny, the only member of my family to visit me by then was Diana. She came for the day and went for a walk around the grounds with me while her husband and two daughters went into Oxford. I went out to the car with her, when they returned to pick her up, to say hello to them. I must have still been on close observations as she was careful to accompany me back to the ward before they left. She gave me wool and crochet hooks, and some little presents from the children.

One evening, when I was feeling sociable enough to sit in the quad with the others, the telephone rang. Someone came to tell Rob that it was for him and he went to take the call. Later he returned, to tell me that my mother was on the telephone for me. I remember being surprised, as I had not heard the second ring. When I spoke to Mother she said nothing about having talked to Rob.

One morning Nick Rose came to me following the ward round and said, 'I understand your mother would like to see me.' I looked blank and told him that it was news to me. He had approached me to ask me how I would like the interview to be conducted. Did I want to be in on all of it or just part of it? I had come to trust Nick so I felt content to say that I would be quite happy with Mother seeing him alone if that was what she wanted.

The appointment was for three o'clock but as time went on there was no sign of Mother. I had to approach Rob to ask if she was clear about the arrangements, since he, so I discovered, knew more than I. He apologised for not having told me but he had quite reasonably assumed that my mother had done so. Anyway, he was able to tell me that my mother had telephoned the ward to find out the arrangements. I wondered what had happened, as Mother was not one to be late for an appointment. When she eventually arrived Dr Rose had had to go into a meeting so was not available. Keith had been waiting for her at Oxford Station but she had had to change twice and all her trains were late, hence her late arrival.

The first thing she said to me was, 'Veronica, I've come to take you home.'

Steve Johnston, the senior house officer (SHO), arrived and suggested that we go into the blue room and start a discussion. We went into the blue room but Mother told him that she was sure he was a very nice doctor but she had arranged to see Dr Rose and she would see Dr Rose. My mother was a very determined person and always went to the top. I found the atmosphere tense so I stood up to go out, using my need for the cup of tea in my room as an excuse. Steve said he really thought I ought to stay but Keith spoke up for me and I went down to my room.

When I came back, Nick had arrived. He went in to talk to my mother and then came out for me a little while later. I went in and he explained that Mother was suggesting that I go back to Salisbury and have treatment as an outpatient. He then told me that they did not think I was ready to leave hospital. He asked me what I wanted. I thought about it, then said, 'Can I have a quiet word?'

The others left the room and Nick and I were alone. He moved his chair closer, knowing that, where I was concerned, a quiet word could be assumed to be just that. I explained that I would rather stay where I was and did not want to go to the Old Manor as an outpatient. Nick asked me if I felt able to say that, or did I want him to. I asked him to. When the others returned, he told them what I wanted and Mother accepted it.

Because of the difficulties Mother had had in her travel from Salisbury, Keith said that he would take her all the way home. Before they left, I was able to go to a village pub with them. I spoke to her, as I did not want her to go home feeling rejected. She had come with my best interests at heart, as ever.

One day Richard visited me. The first thing he said was a declaration: 'I've just had a row with your mother. Since I hate your family and you hate mine, I don't think we can stay together in the long term.'

I was totally shocked and could think of nothing to say. I stood up, with my back to him, and felt an increasing sense of panic. I simply turned around and left the room, went through the quad and out of the building without any of the nursing staff noticing. I did what I had often done when I was very distressed – I walked, and walked and walked. I went down to Sandford Lock, where Rob had taken me on a walk a few days before, crossed the river and went along the riverside path. Apparently two nurses went to the lock, thinking I may have gone there, having been to the lock only a few days before, but by the time they were there I had gone up river and out of sight. It was raining and I was wearing a light cotton summer dress and sandals. The path was turning to mud but I took no notice as my sandals became covered and I kicked the mud up my legs and onto my dress. Soon I was soaked to the skin.

I must have been out for some two or three hours before I began to calm down and decided to retrace my steps. I returned as dusk was falling.

I walked onto the ward and Melanie, a nursing assistant, was the first one to see me. 'Veronica!' she said, in amazement, as well she might, given the state I was in. She put out her hand to me. She took me into the nursing office where Rob, who was in charge that evening, was seated behind the desk. He wiped his hand across his brow and said, 'Veronica! – am I glad to see you! Phew! What a relief!'

I was amazed at the relief with which I was welcomed. I had expected to be greeted with an unenthusiastic, 'Oh, it's you, is it?' As it was I was even further dismayed when Rob picked up the telephone and contacted the police to tell them that I was back. They had been concerned enough to call out the police to look for me.

I heard someone say that Richard was still there, as Steve, the

SHO, came in. I cannot remember what he actually said, but I remember getting the impression that he was trying to 'play it cool'. This irritated me. Did he think I was some child whose naughtiness was best discouraged by being ignored?

Someone got me a cup of tea. I had started to feel cold, soaking wet as I was. Melanie got a blanket and wrapped it around my shoulders. Steve remarked that that was a good idea. Andrea took me to my room.

Andrea was as sweet and kind as ever, getting together some clothes for me and encouraging me to get changed. She asked if I wanted to speak to Richard but I said that I did not, as I did not think that he wanted me anymore. Andrea insisted that he did, adding that he had been very worried about me. Eventually I let her persuade me and we went to the quad. Someone brought me a baked potato saved from tea, but I did not eat it. Richard sat and held my hand. Andrea had been right, he had been very worried, a fact that was later to have repercussions. I was very tearful.

Later, I found it incredible that I had acted in such a manner, running out in such a ridiculous panic. The next day I apologised to Steve and to Rob for causing such concern. Steve commented that it was all right, I had obviously been faced with more than I could cope with. Rob was equally forgiving. I felt very aware that I had caused a lot of trouble and concern, but it still amazed me that they had been so worried about me.

Chapter 9

Off close observations – Visit from SCBU's bereavement counsellor – First visit from work colleagues – Moira visits

---

Richard and I used to go to the BBC Prom concerts every year. We shared a love of classical music. As the time came for the first concert for which we had tickets, I was uncertain whether I could cope with it, enjoyable as the concerts normally were for me. I had asked one of the charge nurses and Steve Johnston and both had unhesitatingly given a positive answer. I remained uncertain, however.

Early one evening I met Nick Rose just as he was about to leave the ward. 'Could you spare me a few minutes?' I asked. He nodded, then lent back against the wall with his arms folded. I told him that I was 'canvassing opinion' about whether I should go to a Prom concert. Nick smiled.

'Shall we find somewhere to sit down?' Nick said.

It was small things like that that made me find it easy to talk to him. There was a suggestion that it was important that we were comfortable so that we could give the subject our full attention. I noticed that he tended to tell me at the beginning of a conversation how much time we had, even if it was just five minutes. I wondered about this but then realised that it meant he could say we would have to finish without my feeling that the termination of the conversation was related to me or to what I was saying.

Even after the two positive responses I had had, I continued to be uncertain. I was not sure whether my reservations reflected an unwillingness that was unjustified – in other words, whether I was making excuses for myself – or whether I had legitimate fears.

Dr Rose, characteristically, did not give an immediate answer. After considering what I had said he asked, 'Is this something you have done before?'

'Oh yes,' I answered. 'We go to the Proms every year.'

'Is it the sort of thing that you would normally enjoy?'

'Yes, I always enjoy classical concerts.'

'How are you going to get there?'

'We drive to Ealing, where we leave the car, then complete the journey on the underground.'

'When would you expect to be back here?'

I thought about it, then said, 'Probably not before eleven o'clock.'

Nick listened carefully to the replies then gave his opinion. 'I don't think you should go this time, though perhaps in a week or so you will be better able to cope with it. What concerns me most is the journey, rather than the concert itself.'

I was actually relieved at this response, apart from anything else it suggested that my personal doubts were justified. I actually did get to three Proms that summer, being allowed to go on condition that Richard stayed with me at all times and that I did not stay out all night.

It was after the conversation about the concert that Nick mentioned the amitriptyline. 'Do you know that the dose has been increased?' he asked.

'No, I don't, no one has told me.'

'The dose is being increased by 25 mg to 175 mg. There is good evidence that even a small increase such as that is often sufficient to bring about a recognisable improvement. We felt that we should do this as your improvement is rather slow.'

I felt irritated that I had heard this news quite fortuitously; as the result of a meeting with Nick when I had stopped him to discuss something entirely different. Communications on the ward were frustratingly bad. Getting a message to the right person was near impossible. If you asked someone a question and they did not know the answer, it was rare that they came back to you.

I gradually began to feel more secure on the ward. I began to relate to the people around me and see them as a source of comfort and support, rather than seeing them as a threat from which I needed to hide. This was a slow process, however. At first matters were complicated by the sort of paranoid fears I would not previously have associated with depression. I described it as feeling as if I were taking part in some elaborate game. It was as though everyone around me were playing the game and had somehow managed to draw me into it. I found myself as a reluctant participant, unable to stop playing the part I had been allocated. It felt as if the people around me had control of me, and were dictating my movements. Was this a reflection of my fear of losing control completely?

Part of me realised that these feelings did not reflect the real situation, yet I sometimes seemed to be struggling to maintain contact with reality. This conflict made it difficult for me to trust the people around me, particularly the nursing staff, who, after all, had ultimate control. They could dictate where I could and could not go. To me there were times when everyone around me seemed unreal – or was it me who was unreal?

Gradually, I became more at ease. As my state of mind improved, I became more responsive. I was able to cope with greater freedom. I went from close observations to 'known whereabouts', which meant that I had to tell the staff where I was going and when I would be back. Whether my plans were agreed to was up to the discretion of the nursing staff. At first, I found even this degree of freedom disconcerting and anxiety provoking.

On one occasion I was hovering around the open side door. I felt untrusting of myself and unsafe. Tim came to get something from the medical office. He went up to me with a parcel and gave it to me. I looked at it, then commented that it was from my sister Diana, as I recognised the writing.

'Is she a nurse as well?' Tim asked.

'Yes, how did you know?'

Tim pointed to the parcel and I realised that it was sealed with surgical tape. Diana must have packed it up while working one night. I thought it probable that it was a birthday present but did not mention that as I did not want anyone to know my birthday was coming up.

Having Tim there, I decided to express my anxiety about being alone and my feelings of insecurity.

'Well, you have been used to someone being with you at all times,' he commented.

'I don't think I trust myself on my own. I feel as if I might go away,' I answered. 'I don't feel as if there is anything wrong with me. I just feel that I can't cope,' I added.

'When I look at you, I see someone showing all the signs of an illness called depression,' Tim replied.

'I feel unsafe.'

'Being on your own might well make you feel vulnerable. Why don't you come down the other end where everyone else is?' he suggested, after we had discussed it. 'Perhaps you could think about how much support you need to feel safe. It may be that you need closer watching for a while.'

I thought about it carefully after Tim had left me in the quad. Every day, all day, for over a fortnight, I had had a nurse with me. There had been no opportunity for me to leave the hospital premises and put myself in danger. I felt as if something heavy, that perhaps I had been carrying for some time, had been lifted from me. It felt as if something substantial was missing, a burden, but an important burden, something that had seemed to weigh on me while it was there but that I felt strange without. It gave me freedom, but perhaps too great a freedom.

After lunch I found Tim. 'I think I would feel better if I had someone with me, for a couple more days,' I confessed. 'After that, I will try to behave myself.'

'I don't see it as your misbehaving,' Tim said, with serious disapproval. 'You are unwell and if you need that sort of support you should have it. If you had a broken leg, I would not take away your crutches.'

Gradually I began to improve and this was reflected in my behaviour. I spent more time in the quad, more time in the company of other people. I found the courage to speak in groups, even in the dreaded community meetings, although I relied on someone's eliciting a response from me; it was a long time before I was able to make an unsolicited comment. On one occasion there was a discussion in the community meeting about why some patients never attended. One of the nurses said that they probably found such a big meeting difficult. Dr Rose remarked, 'Yes, but Veronica finds it difficult yet she makes a determined effort to be here,' commenting on my presence. I was amazed at this praise for my pathetic efforts.

I even began to go for walks around the grounds by myself.

The day before my birthday, Emma came to my room with a florist's box. I opened it and found it full of carnations. There was a card inside. On it was written 'Happy Birthday'. It was from Katherine and Nicholas. Emma said, 'I didn't know it was your birthday.'

'It's not, it's tomorrow,' I answered. I hoped that no one would make a fuss about it.

The next morning Rob came to my room and gave me a card and two wrapped parcels. Inside were a box of Roses chocolates and some lavender talc. The card was signed by those members of

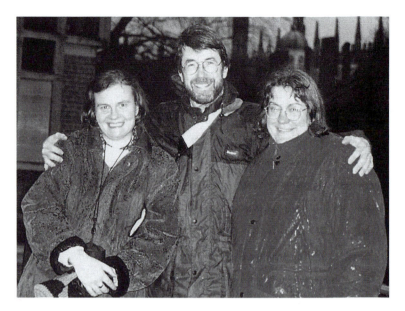

Figure 9.1 With Katherine and Nicholas, in Cambridge.

staff who were there that morning, or the evening before. At tea time there was a large Black Forest gâteau sent up from the kitchen because it was my birthday, of which I had two pieces. Well, it was my birthday.

That evening I went out for the first time. I had asked Nick, explaining that it was my birthday, and that Richard and I were planning to spend the evening with friends. I took with me the present Diana had sent, as yet unopened, and one that Richard had given me.

It felt quite peculiar to get into the car and leave the hospital. At first it made my head spin, mainly, I thought, because of the drugs.

When we arrived, Nicholas was bathing their infant daughter, Sarah. I went into the bathroom and Sarah greeted me with a delighted smile. She then stood up in the bath, pulled out the plug and started to climb out. I felt very flattered to be made so welcome.

We had a quiet but very enjoyable evening. The parcel from Diana contained a lovely cotton summer dress that she had made for me. When I wore it on the ward, I had several complimentary comments about it. I was often complimented on my clothes and on how I looked, by patients, staff and visitors. It was nice, though it rather surprised me. Richard gave me some earrings, the first time he had ever bought me jewellery. The signs were that the situation was beginning to overwhelm him, but I think he was trying to show that he still loved me, even if things were not going so well.

It was not until close to the time of my discharge that I was able to go to my own home for the weekend. It felt very strange to walk into the house again. What I most noticed was the smell of an ordinary domestic home – carpets, curtains, soft furnishings. I never noticed it so strongly again.

As my discharge approached, I was able to go out for a drink when Clare and Keith visited in the evening.

Initially I had not wanted to communicate with anyone from my workplace. My sense of failure was centred on my work and my professional status as a nurse. I began to realise that I would have to make contact at some point. During the first few weeks of my hospital stay, I had received several messages to say that someone from work had telephoned to ask how I was. I remembered one message in particular. It was from the unit's bereavement counsellor, Jenni, who had left her telephone number in case I wanted to contact her. When I considered getting in touch with someone from work, it was Jenni I thought of as the best person to contact initially. This was partly because of her personal qualities and partly because she worked on SCBU in her capacity as a nursery nurse (but in the 'cold' nursery, not in the area in which I usually worked – intensive care).

One evening Jenni came to visit me. She brought with her an arrangement of flowers from Moira's garden, put in a small basket. Jenni also gave me a large card signed by everyone at work. I did not open it until after she had gone.

Jenni ran a post-natal depression group for which she had reported to Nick Rose, before he had left for Oxford, so I assumed that she would know who I referred to when I said, 'My consultant is someone you will know.' Jenni simply looked puzzled, so I said, 'Nick Rose.'

'Oh Veronica, he's lovely!' Jenni responded when she heard his name.

Jenni left and I was alone in my room. It was then that I opened the card she had brought. There were a lot of messages, mostly about the absence of Radio Three on the unit, or their missing my technical skills. There was one message in particular that surprised me, one of the larger messages. It said 'Hurry up and get well quickly because we miss you and need you' and came from one of the unit's consultants. There were lots of other messages on the card. I found myself glad to have it.

I still found it difficult to cope with the idea of any of my nursing colleagues from the unit coming to visit me. The first time they did, I found myself becoming very tense in anticipation. To cope, I was inclined to take chlorpromazine. (Tim had got the prescription changed to a 'prn' – taken as needed – dose and I occasionally took one to help me through a difficult morning.) Karen, however, helped me to cope by getting me to lie on my bed and use relaxation techniques, while one of her scented candles burned in the room. When my colleagues arrived, she sat them down and gave them a cup of tea so that I had a little more time to get myself together. The visit was by no means the ordeal that I had assumed it would be and subsequent visits by work colleagues did not cause me such anxiety.

The first time I actually went out of the hospital gates, I was with two other patients and Melanie. I was still under close observation and felt quite anxious at leaving the protective confines of the hospital. Although Melanie was careful to keep me near her, I still felt rather anxious. We went to the village shops. It all seemed quite weird, for previously it had seemed as if the hospital existed in a vacuum.

Once the level of supervision that I received was lessened, I began to use the freedom it allowed, though with some uncertainty initially. I began to go for walks around the hospital grounds and my confidence gradually improved.

Eventually I was able to move to the other corridor where the fire escape opened onto the courtyard, and which was always open in good weather. The rooms were nicer, less like prison cells. They had normal sash windows and overlooked a lawn with a beautiful mature weeping willow tree in the centre. I was lucky to have a double room again. This time there was another bed in it but I was assured that I would not have to share.

It was after I had moved to that room that Jenni visited again. Rob came to my door and gave me a message that the person who was due to visit would be bringing a colleague. He could not tell me who it was. I wondered if it was Moira.

Jenni arrived and came to my room on her own. She sat down and explained that Moira was with her but had stayed in the car. After we had had a chat we could go out to see her, if I felt I wanted to. This, I thought, was as near an admission of guilt in regard to me that I would ever get from Moira. She had never admitted that she had been in any way wrong in her professional relationship with me, but if that were indeed the case, it seemed an odd way for her to behave.

The way Jenni put the idea of my seeing Moira gave me a choice – I suspected that there was some degree of uncertainty about whether I would agree to see her. I had commented to Nick Rose only recently that I felt Moira thought I had a confidence that was unassailable. I really thought that she was amazed when it became so obvious that the strain was too much for me. I seemed to be a peculiar combination of apparent strength hiding a very real vulnerability. I thought that Moira considered that, because I was technically able and generally efficient, and presumably knew it, I would be able to withstand any amount of criticism. I had often felt angry about it. What right had anyone to assume that I was immune to criticism, to ignore my feelings, not to respect my view? Had anyone the right to act upon the assumption that I cared less than others about how I was treated? Did my feelings count for less because I was apparently good at my job?

Of course I did go out to see Moira.

Jenni and Moira came back to my room with me. They talked for a while. I, however, still had feelings of anger towards Moira and could not yet fully forgive her. I was angry about the way that she had failed me as my senior manager. I thought that I had a right to expect some support from her, as did the rest of the staff, including the nursery nurses, who had received scant sympathy. She had been totally disloyal to her staff. I did not think that there was any point in harbouring resentment about it, yet I knew that I had some way to go before I could overcome it. I hoped that, in time, I would feel better about it. From where I was then, however, it was hard to feel very positive, struggling as I was to deal with the resultant problems.

Meanwhile, I thought, I must try to find something constructive in all this mess. I am sure that turning around and blaming others is not constructive, though perhaps a properly expressed anger is understandable and therapeutic.

We talked a while about nothing in particular, carefully avoiding anything that was at all serious, let alone what had happened between us on SCBU. Jenni did, however, invite Moira to look at the card I had received from my colleagues, drawing her attention to the consultant's message that had made such an impression on me. Moira read it and expressed her amazement that the consultant had written such a message. I wondered what she really thought, as that consultant had been highly supportive of my going ahead to appeal.

Chapter 10

Difficulties in community meetings – Reg responds to my distress – Tim intervenes after distressing meeting – Appointments with Nick

I had very much begun to come out of myself. I still felt very uncertain, and my feelings on many things were ambivalent. I did not want to rely too much on others, yet I felt the need for encouragement and support. I was afraid of becoming too comfortable in the patient role, but also afraid that leaving hospital would leave me exposed and unable to cope. I wondered where responsibility for myself ended and began to feel unreasonably guilty about what I could not be expected to achieve. I did not know where to set my parameters anymore. There were too many questions and not enough answers. I did not know how to judge myself, how to sort out right from wrong.

The situation was improving, however, especially where the groups were concerned. Although the community group remained problematic, I felt happier in the women's group and the small group.

One morning someone raised the subject in the community meeting of how safe people felt there. One patient responded by standing up, declaring 'I'll show you how safe I feel,' and walking out.

I was asked how I felt about the patient's action. 'I find it very . . . unsettling,' I answered. In fact I felt quite angry with the woman who had made such a dramatic gesture when I was putting all the effort I could into staying in the room until the end of the meeting. I had never yet walked out of a group and I did not want to do so then. When I thought about it though, it seemed to me that walking out of the room in that way was counterproductive – it could not fail to bring attention to oneself. I even wondered whether this was part of the purpose of standing up and dramatically marching out. You do not behave like that, I thought, if you did not want to attract attention to yourself. What really upset me about the situation was that I was left feeling abandoned and alone after the meeting had finished. All the nurses disappeared into a feedback session. I wandered about feeling rather reluctant, vulnerable as I was, to go outside and walk, for my inclination when distressed was to go outside and walk and keep on walking.

Eventually I did go outside, by which time I was crying and obviously distressed. As I walked towards the hospital gates, I heard a voice calling my name. I turned away from the path and made my way across the lawn, in order to avoid whoever had called. The person came up to me and began to walk by my side. I felt like shouting 'Go away, who asked you to interfere?' As he walked beside me, I realised that the person was Reg, a manic depressive who was visiting the ward at the time, though he was not an inpatient. Reg would not be put off when I turned away and changed direction. He simply kept with me. He kept by me and started to talk to me. 'Now don't go out there, stay in the grounds,' he said when we reached the gates. He steered me clear and began to walk towards the extensive lawns.

I walked around the gardens with Reg for almost an hour. He kept by me, chatting all the time. Despite myself, I began to feel grateful for his evident care and concern. When he had first approached me, he had been going for a bus which only came hourly, but he did not go to catch it until he had delivered me safely back to the ward.

Reg always had his personal stereo with him. 'What music do you like?' he asked me.

'Classical music,' I answered.

'Oh, classical eh? I haven't heard any of that,' he replied. A couple of weeks later Reg approached me on the ward and told me that he had bought a cassette of classical music. 'I find some of it quite enjoyable,' he admitted. Eventually, however, he gave the tape to me.

'You must let me give you something for it,' I told him.

'Oh, no, no, I don't want anything for it, all I want is to see you get better,' he replied.

The other time I had difficulties in a community meeting it also involved Reg, though on this occasion he was the main source of the discord. Given his earlier behaviour towards me, I could not bring myself to blame him too far. He was somewhat manic that day and displayed a lot of anger, particularly towards Steve Johnston, who was present. The whole situation became very tense, so much so that I made straight for the doors once the meeting finished. Feeling under stress, I, as ever, wanted to go outside. I went directly to the open fire escape. Once more someone called me back, causing me to hesitate. It was Tim, who came up to me. 'I was feeling quite tense in that meeting,' he admitted, 'so much so that I felt concerned for how you might be feeling. Look, will you come back inside with me?'

We went to the blue room. 'I want to go outside,' I told him.

'Yes, I can understand that but I would rather you had someone with you.' Tim looked around thoughtfully, obviously at something of a loss to know who he could send with me. 'I appreciate why you want to go outside but I would really rather you did not go on your own, especially since you are obviously distressed. Wait a minute, I know. Come with me.' We went into the quad and Tim approached a trainee priest who was spending some time on the unit. He happily agreed to accompany me. As we were about to go, Tim said, 'And don't go near any cars, all right?'

What made the difference between the two events was Tim's sensitivity to the way I felt as a result of the meeting. Previously all the nurses had just disappeared into a feedback meeting; this time, Tim appreciated my response and my desire to go outside. His comment about the cars was an expression of concern for my safety, not an order. During the second meeting, I had said nothing. It was perhaps ironic that it was following the first meeting, during which I had made a difficult attempt to express my response, that the nurses had failed to appreciate my reaction.

Of the medical staff, I continued to find Nick Rose the most sensitive and easy to talk to. I once heard Karen say of him, 'Charm's his middle name, but he can be quite firm about what he wants.' Rob commented to me, 'Sometimes he's so gentle that I want to protect him.'

Steve was always pleasant and helpful, but I did not have as much faith in him. He saw me and Richard together a few times to try and improve Richard's understanding of my illness and to help with the difficulties we had between us. Nigel did not have the gentle approach of his consultant but I came to respect his judgement, although I still felt that he had been wrong over the ECT question. I thought that an attempt to give me ECT against my will would have been potentially disastrous. To say that the treatment would have had such an effect that I would have realised the decision was the right one seemed too trite an answer in the circumstances.

On those occasions when I wanted to discuss something with Nick, I would ask the staff to pass the message on and he invariably sought me out some time on that day. Once I asked Karen to pass on a message to Nick Rose, saying that I would like to see him. Karen suggested that I see his secretary to make an appointment and took me upstairs to his office. The next time I asked Nick if I could see him, he suggested that I make an appointment with his secretary. I went upstairs again; I was impressed by the fact that the secretary remembered me and my name. She had only seen me once before, when I had been with Karen. After that, I would usually see Nick in his office. 'Office' did not quite seem to be the right word. It was a large room connecting through to his secretary's room. The desk and chair were pushed aside in a corner under the window. The main part of the room was taken up by upholstered chairs with batik drapes.

I wondered if I were taking up too much of his time, yet he would inevitably end a session by telling me to make another appointment with Joy, his secretary, if I needed to. I supposed that he would not have said that if I were being a nuisance.

By the time I was coming up to discharge in September, I was allowed to go where and when I wanted, including down to the village shops, or for a walk along by the river. I had been to three Proms concerts with Richard and spent a weekend at home. I discussed with Karen how I would get my confidence back in driving, although I did not feel that I would have many problems there. I had always enjoyed driving and had passed my advanced driving test. However, I was surprised to find that my leg shook as I put it on the pedal. It was not long before I calmed down though, and was able to take the car out. I was glad about that, as we lived in a village and I needed the car if I was to have any freedom or independence.

Of course, one may wonder what had happened to make me ready for discharge. Later events established that my medication regime was not as effective as had been hoped. However, I certainly improved. Being taken into hospital removed the necessity of coping with the usual demands of life. I had no doubt just reached the stage, at the time of my admission, of being quite unable to cope with work. Hospital took that, by then unbearable, strain from me. It also took away the responsibility of feeding myself. For months before my admission, I had been surviving on drinking chocolate and biscuits precisely because I lacked the incentive or ability to keep myself alive. As a result, I had lost a great deal of weight. Once I was admitted, I no longer had any responsibility for providing my own nutrition – meals arrived on the ward three times a day and all I had to do was to choose from the selection. It also cushioned me from other responsibilities of life, such as finance. Hospital provided me with a haven in which so many things that would have concerned me were absent.

In addition, depression is not curable – you can simply attempt to control it until it goes into a spontaneous remission. On some occasions this may have been what was happening.

One of the most important responsibilities that hospital took from me was that of my personal safety. One of the main reasons I tolerated later admissions was that I came to regard Phoenix as my safe place. At home, before my admission, I had gone through agonising periods when my mind was persuading me that I should destroy myself. Once I was in hospital, others took responsibility for my safety.

There were other positive things about being on the ward. These were mainly represented by the role of the staff – Nick Rose, the nurses and therapists – who encouraged me to be positive about myself when all seemed entirely negative. The nurses were the ones who were with you day and night. Time spent with a caring and sensitive nurse could be very helpful as well as comforting. A good 'named' nurse – that is, one who had a responsibility for particular patients – was often important in encouraging my understanding and building on what little self-confidence I had. At least part of my self-regard had to be rekindled before I could claim any form of recovery. Later events showed, however, that this was something that was very fragile.

Also, there were the different groups, the small group and the women's group, the therapeutic groups such as drama group and art group.

All these different things worked to restore my fragile self-regard and gave me time and freedom simply to recover.

Chapter 11 ▬▬

Discharge – Richard goes away overnight – My reaction –
Second admission – Sister's wedding in Salisbury

I was discharged on Wednesday, 20 September 1989, exactly two
months after my admission. Evening handover for the staff had
just finished when Richard arrived, so it must have been about nine
o'clock. We put my bags in the back of the car, with Richard saying
very little. I wondered if something was wrong. I said goodbye to the
nurses and we left. Richard said nothing on the way back. He drove
up the motorway at 90 mph – I could see the speedometer. Being
driven at speed would not usually have bothered me. That night,
however, it made me feel anxious and scared. Richard's moroseness
did not help.

When we got home I went straight in and sat down, visibly
shaking. Richard brought the bags in. He then told me that I ought
to go to Salisbury, as he did not want to be responsible for me. He
said that he could never be sure what I might do – alluding to the
time when I had gone along the river and Rob had informed Oxford
police, I suspected. I was very stressed, and quite stunned.

I had been in the house for two nights and one day when, on
Friday morning, Richard told me not to expect him home that day,

as he was going somewhere after work and would be staying all night.

I was deeply upset. Why was he behaving in this manner? It was so sad that we could not work together to cope with all these problems, but I think that we each needed the other to help us to cope in a situation that neither of us knew how to handle. Richard had always been so affectionate and protective towards me, and it was not really in his nature to be cruel, but I felt he was being so.

I was due to spend that day at Phoenix. When I arrived, I met Tim coming out of the nursing office. He stopped and asked me how things had gone. I could not say anything. I looked at the floor and shook my head, confused by my emotions and unable to express them. Tim put his hand on my shoulder sympathetically, then said decisively, 'Coffee.' He took me into the office and made me a cup of coffee, then went away, leaving me with the others in the office. I cannot remember who was there.

When Tim returned, he asked me if I had an appointment to see anyone. I said no. He suggested that we go to the blue room where I could tell him about it.

I told Tim what had happened. When we had stopped talking, I sat wringing my hands, tense and distressed. 'I feel as if I want to cry, but I can't.'

'Yes, I can see that,' Tim responded. 'Would a hug help?' I nodded and he put his arm around my shoulders and gave me a hug. The fact that someone was prepared to come so close was a great comfort when Richard had so distanced himself.

I needed medication to take out (TTOs) but no one could be found to write them up. I had decided to go to Nicholas and Katherine, to the house in Witney to which they had moved when I was in hospital. I said that I would return to collect my drugs. Tim had expressed concern at Richard's going and leaving me alone overnight.

I went back to find that my TTOs were ready. I was seated in the office when Steve Johnson came in. He asked another patient present to leave and closed the door. I once again went over what had happened. I was tearful by then, and very distressed. This was made worse by the fact that Steve did not seem to believe me. I got the impression that he thought that I was not telling the whole truth. I must have done or said something to induce Richard to behave the way he had. 'This is indicative of something, Veronica!' he said. I felt bad enough without his taking that line. If he found it hard to believe, how did he think I felt?

While he was speaking, the telephone rang so he answered it. It was Katherine checking that I had got there safely. She said that if I needed somewhere to stay, I could always go to them. She later told me that she had considered how she would feel if Nick had said to her what Richard had said to me.

There was general concern about my staying on my own in the house overnight. They accepted the suggestion that I should go to Arborfield and stay with Clare and Keith. I arrived on their doorstep late that night and they were happy for me to stay. Over the next few days they became used to my turning up at odd times, despite which they were always welcoming.

I am not really very clear about what happened during the next two weeks. Karen said that she was worried about my indecisiveness. Nick commented that my moving about from place to place concerned him. These were certainly aspects of that time. I think they reflected the shock and confusion that I felt as a reaction to Richard's rejection of me. The first discharge might have worked if I had made sufficient effort and had gone home to some degree of support and stability. The situation had been radically altered when I was not sent home to the expected situation. I was in no way prepared to cope with the actual situation I found myself in, or the difficulties I was faced with.

One day I was in Phoenix when I went out to my car, distressed and crying. I passed another patient and I suspect that it was he who told Mike, the nurse in charge that day. He came out, opened the door and, sitting back on his heels, and commented, 'I can see you're very upset.' I cannot remember what else was said; the next thing I can remember was standing in the A6 corridor with Mike talking to me. 'Veronica, you've got to take some steps forward at some stage.' My response to that was to walk out. I was obviously not in the mood to listen to simple truth.

I went outside and leant beside the wall. It was just going dark. I felt like going on one of my foot tours of Oxford. My car would be sitting outside the hospital – they might get worried? No, they would not, I thought. From what Mike had said, he knew that I was very distressed, but basically in my right mind, unlike those times when I had been an inpatient and escaped the ward. Anyway, I admitted to myself, they deserved better from me than childish and irresponsible gestures. I decided that I must go in and say that I would be going to Clare's and I must find Mike to say it to. So that is what I did, as much as a penance as to give information.

One morning I spoke to one of the nurses on the telephone and tried to express my confusion over where to go and what to do. Steve telephoned and said that he thought I could cope. I did not have much faith in Steve by now, for all I could remember was his scepticism when I had told him what had happened when I had gone home. I asked to see Nick Rose and Steve readily agreed, signifying that he was not as sure about the situation as his advice suggested.

I went to Phoenix on a Monday morning and Steve told me that he had arranged for me to see Dr Rose at 11.00, on 9 October 1989. When Nick arrived, we went into the blue room with Steve and Karen. I described how I had felt like crashing the car. While going along the A40 I had actually gone as far as to identify a spot where I could go off the road, where I would go into a field and so not involve other people. It had not lasted long, and the fact that I came across an accident on the other carriageway brought me around to normality. It was an isolated moment, not the persistent 'you ought kill yourself' compulsion that so plagued me when I was very depressed.

Nick questioned me closely and in detail about my behaviour over the weekend and how I had felt. He suggested that I should be commenced on lithium and should come into hospital while it was started. He had mentioned lithium, a mood stabiliser, before. It could be quickly and impressively effective. The problem was that there is a narrow therapeutic/toxic ratio, meaning that the blood level required for therapeutic levels was close to the level that will cause toxicity. For this reason, blood levels of lithium need to be measured frequently when being introduced and about three-monthly once an optimum level is established.

'You seem to have lost confidence,' Nick remarked.

Karen took me to the office and told me what rooms were free in the A6 corridor and I chose the double one I had been in before. I gave the keys to my car to Karen once I had removed what I wanted.

I was feeling vulnerable and Phoenix was a safe place for me. But I also had an immense sense of defeat. I felt as if the stuffing had been knocked out of me. It was not the sense of defeat resulting from the conviction of worthlessness that is so much a part of deep depression. This defeatism was not irrational or impervious to reason; this was genuine, this was real – I had no cocoon of introspection to cushion me in an unreal world of my own. I felt exposed and, although I thought that I should have been able to manage without re-admission, I was glad enough to be there whatever the cause. Yet I felt like an impostor, as if I should not have been there.

The research nurse, Ali, came to see me. They were investigating lithium in the research department that was above Phoenix. She had got Dr Rose's permission to include me if I agreed. She explained what my participation would entail and gave me the requisite piece of paper so that I would have it in writing. My participation would mean a delay in starting lithium, as baseline observations would have to be established. I would initially need to go upstairs to have a heart reading or electrocardiogram (ECG), and my height and weight recorded. Following that, I would have a session in the research department. This would have to take place before I could be commenced on lithium. However, after the initial session it was decided to continue at the research department at the Warneford, the hospital at which I had attended outpatients that July.

On the Wednesday night, before the first proper research session at the Warneford, I was not given any of my drugs, though apparently this was not necessary. It did mean that I did not get much sleep the night before. On the Thursday morning, I was standing in the room next to the medical office waiting for Ali. I did not feel right, though I could not have explained what exactly was wrong. One thing I did know was that I did not want to go across town to another hospital. Mike and Tim were in the nearby clinical room and I felt like going over and saying, 'don't let her take me away'. Ali arrived, friendly and pleasant, nevertheless someone I hardly knew.

It was peculiar to feel myself at the Warneford again. When I had first been there, I had not raised my eyes from the floor, so nothing I saw was familiar. The research department was obviously new to me. Ali weighed me then asked me to get on a hospital bed where I sat, leaning against the pillows. I took the clipboard, pen and two forms that she asked me to fill in. One was the Beck Inventory – a familiar way of measuring a patient's level of depression, as Vivienne, the psychologist at Phoenix gave me one before each session with her. The second was a series of statements to which I had to answer true or false. As I filled it in, I became aware that I was responding 'true' to every negative statement and 'false' to every positive. Very clever, I thought, who was responsible for this? I had that feeling again, as if I were being drawn into some strange game, I didn't know how to play. In that room in the Warneford, I felt alone and vulnerable.

Ali seemed to realise that there was something wrong and was kind and sympathetic, as was the doctor who came in to put a needle in my vein. Ali asked what drugs I had been given the night before and was surprised when I said I had not been given any. I asked if it would affect the results. She reassured me but said that she was concerned that the lack of drugs had obviously affected me.

When I arrived back with Ali, about two hours later, I walked straight down to my room. There was a knock on the door and Tim came in. He sat on his heels in front of me, sat on the bed. I told him that I did not realise how awful I had felt until I had done those questionnaires. 'Would a hug help?' he asked. When I nodded, he sat beside me and put his arm around me. Rob had once said that before coming to Phoenix, Tim had worked on a unit where, more than was usual, they employed touch and physical contact to convey sympathy and give comfort. I was not surprised.

Tim suggested that I might feel better with people near and I agreed to go to the quad. He said that he would feel happier with me there. I went into the office. Linda made me a cup of tea, but I drank only a little of it. When I walked to my room, Linda followed me and asked me to return to the office or the quad.

I was in the office when Steve sat down with a casual air. However, when another patient came in he asked her to leave because he wanted to have a word with me. I can remember little of the ensuing conversation, except that he tried to persuade me that I was too unwell to go to my youngest sister's wedding. With my eyes to the floor, I did not see him leave. I glanced up as the door was pushed open. It was Nigel Courtenay. He asked me to come to the blue room. I was puzzled by all this. Apparently I had scored very highly on the Beck Inventory hopelessness scale and the doctor at the Warneford had warned Phoenix that I was at high risk of suicide.

He asked me how I was feeling. I told him that it was as if a switch had been flicked. 'And when it was flicked, what effect did it have?' I answered that it made me feel as if I were taking part in some elaborate game. It seemed as if things around me were not real. I was confused.

Dr Courtenay said that they would have to see how the lithium affected me, otherwise ECT might have to be considered. It seems strange that I did not respond to that. I really felt as if I did not care. He wrote in my notes that he was sure the doctor at the Warneford was right about my being deeply depressed and at risk of suicide.

We then got onto the subject of Eleanor's wedding, in Salisbury that coming Saturday, 14 October 1989. I said that I intended to go; in fact, I insisted that I 'have to go'. He told me that I did not have to go, that he was sure my sister would understand. It seemed to me that he did not understand – I had to go, there was no question about it, I had to go and I would go.

Eventually it was decided that a decision on the matter would be made the next day, when it would be arranged for a member of my family to come to speak to him or Nick Rose.

I was better the next day. Whether this was me rousing myself, a coincidental change in mood, or that I had had my medication the previous night, I do not know. It was Clare who came and met with me and Nick. He asked Clare what it would involve. She said there would be the ceremony, followed by a reception in a hotel with a disco in the evening. The result of the conversation was that Nick Rose was prepared to let me go if I felt that I could cope with it but I was not to drive. As usual, Nick preferred to let me push myself if I could, provided I observed certain conditions. Clare and I left saying that I would be back on Sunday.

I already had something to wear. When I had been at Clare's one weekend she had taken me into a shop in Wokingham and pointed out two outfits for me to try on. I had chosen a suit and had bought a hat to match it. When I took the wedding photographs to Phoenix, Liz saw one of me holding my baby niece, with my young nephew, Stephen. 'Who's that?' she asked.

Katherine said, 'You look incredibly elegant. It's amazing!' Apparently I did not look myself when dressed up.

I stayed with Peter and Sheila over that weekend. I went to the service and to the reception, having asked Eleanor and Stephen if

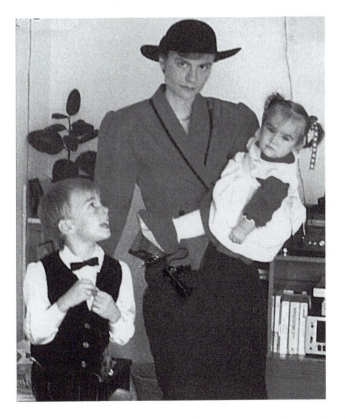

Figure 11.1 Me holding my baby niece, with my young nephew, on the day of Eleanor and Stephen's wedding.

I could change the seating a little so that I was beside close members of my family. I felt more secure with that arrangement. I decided that I would not go to the disco but have a quiet evening on my own. Pete was concerned about my spending the evening on my own but I reassured him.

I returned on the Sunday as arranged. On Monday morning I was seated in the quad, as those attending the ward round went through to the blue room. Nigel Courtenay asked me how I had managed. I said that I had gone to the service and reception, but not to the disco, adding that I would not normally be inclined to go far for a disco. He gave a slight laugh and said, 'Quite'.

Nick Rose walked through the quad at his usual brisk pace. (I once told Deborah that I was trying to catch Nick Rose. 'Now that's a difficult one – the only way to catch him is to put out your foot when he's passing.') Nick paused, turned and came over to me, asking me how I had got on at the weekend. I told him that I had gone to the service and the reception. 'So you got there with your usual determination,' he commented.

Chapter 12 ▬

Australia – Fears before going – Return to work – Carlisle
to visit my brother – Stop driving on hard shoulder – Third
admission – Nick Rose's visit

For some time my father had been trying to persuade me to go to
Australia with him to visit his brother. It all seemed too adventurous
to me, but I was eventually persuaded to go following my second
discharge. The last time I saw Vivienne, the psychologist who saw
me for cognitive behavioural therapy (CBT), before we went I told
her that I was sure something awful was going to happen while I
was in Australia, and became quite distressed about it. She advised
me to talk to Nick Rose. While I explained it to him I became
increasingly disturbed, rocking in my chair, wringing my hands and
looking at the floor.

I told him that something awful would happen to someone close
to me. I said, 'And when it does it will be *my* fault.'

Nick leant forward and, speaking quietly and calmly as he always
did when I was very upset, asked, 'Do you think that you will be in
some way involved?'

I shook my head. 'I don't think so, not necessarily. But when it does, it will be *my fault*,' was my anguished reply.

Nick leaned back and considered.

'I think I'm going mad,' I said.

Nick leant towards me again and, in his usual calm, quiet way asked, 'What is the worst thing that could happen while you are away?'

I stopped rocking and looked sideways at him. I felt surprised. It was as if he, a sensible and informed person, had revealed a rational element in my crazy idea – perhaps it was not quite so insane an idea after all. 'What I'm afraid of, I suppose.' Here was a connection, a bridge between sanity and insanity.

Nick told me that he did not think my fears were mad, but understandable in the circumstances. 'I think we've underestimated the difficulties this trip will mean for you.' After a pause he said, 'What do you think about going?'

I paused, then answered, 'I've *got* to go.'

Nick accepted this. When I became determined to do something, he was always prepared to support me.

I stayed in Australia for four weeks, spending the Christmas of 1989 there. My father stayed for a month after me but I found that I could not cope with being so far from home for too long. I made the excuse that I had to get back to work.

On Monday, 17 February 1990, I started work again after an absence of seven months. As arranged, I only worked in the cold nursery to start with and then only three and a half days a week. I found my colleagues on SCBU very supportive. As I went around the hospital, I would meet people who would remark that they had not seen me in a long while. People were generally very welcoming.

Fortunately they were going through a quiet time on SCBU. I found things very difficult at first. I had little confidence in my ability to do my job, which was a feeling unknown to me and very difficult to handle. There were times when I had to ask someone else to take over from me, explaining frankly, 'I can't do it, my hands are too shaky.' I saw little point in being anything other than honest. I did not know how much the student midwives knew about me, though there were occasions when they clearly thought that I had not been there long. They expressed surprise when I told them that I had worked there for four years, as they had not seen me during their first secondment to SCBU. I simply explained that I had been on sick leave.

I thought of how confident I used to be and, indeed, how inspiring of confidence in those around me. I had had good relations with almost all the house officers who served on SCBU. They were usually happy to ask for my guidance when appropriate.

Just after the gradings had been announced, I was in the kitchen and had remarked to a colleague that I was thinking of leaving. A junior house officer was there and said, 'Oh, don't go before I've done my senior post.' On my return I lacked all confidence, yet previously, along with certain other members of the nursing staff, I had been used to the doctors relying on us for help and advice. Even the consultants had trusted my judgement.

During the first few weeks at work, I had difficulties with anxiety and a panicky desire to get away. I solved the problem by going into the sitting room with a cup of coffee, allowing myself a given time, ten or fifteen minutes, then going back to the nursery at the end of that time. It was all very difficult though, and very tiring. Although I was sleeping better, I was still not sleeping well.

At this time I was staying with my cousin in Thame while I was working, then going to Salisbury to stay with Mother when not working. Mother was supportive – she knew what it was like to be depressed.

On my return from Australia, I discovered that Katherine and Nicholas had a baby boy born by emergency caesarean section on Christmas Eve. Katherine and baby John were home by the time of my return, although both of them had been quite ill after the birth, which was why they had not let me know their news. John had been nursed on the neonatal unit that I had worked on to get my SCBU qualification. I often went to Witney to see them on my travels.

One weekend I went to see some friends from Durham. Richard had been to see them a few weeks before and had told them that it was his fault we had split up.

In between seeing Nick Rose I continued to see Vivienne. My sessions with her tended to be more emotional than those with Nick. Sometimes I was in tears and had to stay in the room by myself after our meeting, to compose myself. I felt my reaction was inevitable as we concentrated on my emotional responses to things that had happened in the past and how they had affected me. At times I felt angry and frustrated, with a sense of futility. I could not change what had happened in the past, either in my childhood or in the recent past. I said one day that I did not see how I could have avoided what had happened during the last year. Put in the same position, I could not see how I could have behaved differently. Vivienne agreed that there was perhaps nothing else I could have done. This was important to me as it suggested that what I had done could not be assumed to be wrong because of its repercussions. There was the possibility that my reactions had not simply been wrong – my view of the situation, I thought, might actually be defensible. Vivienne was invariably understanding and tolerant of my feelings, though there were actually times when I did not want to be understood, or at least I thought I did not deserve to be so treated, and felt uncomfortable with others' sympathetic responses. Vivienne and Nick treated me with gentle understanding, yet they each did so in a different way. Dr Rose's attitude seemed to derive from a natural compassion. Vivienne's was more in the sense of a simple acknowledgement of the limitations of the state I was in; a recognition that removed from me the onerous obligation of attempting to avoid those limitations. The first time I saw her, during my first admission, Vivienne gave me a short article. She asked me to read it, adding that she would understand if I could not read it all. It seemed to me that she always limited her expectations, accepting that my standard of performance was unavoidably compromised. That made me feel relieved, as I was never being asked to achieve the impossible. But it also made me feel uncomfortable and guilty in accepting the limitations. There were times when I felt that Vivienne should be more forceful, demand better of me, punish me for my weakness by being harsh. She never did, though.

Vivienne helped me make sense of the crazy situation while Nick was invariably encouraging and supportive, always making me feel saner.

In March, Patrick, my brother, had an eye operation for congenital cataracts. Initially the news was very good: he could read the credits on the television. Everyone was delighted to hear of his progress. However, he soon began to suffer complications which threatened to considerably reduce the effectiveness of the eye that had been operated on. It began to look as if he might need another operation. I felt desperately concerned, a concern heightened by my tendency to become anxious when depressed.

At work, Moira took me into the office and asked how I was doing. Not very well was the answer. (Moira never took me aside when things were going well.) I explained about Patrick's operation. I was also affected at the time by the death of my brother-in-law's mother. This I felt vicariously rather than personally – I knew that Diana, her husband and the children were very upset by it.

Moira remarked, 'It keeps on piling up, doesn't it?' It certainly seemed that way. She also commented that I had not spoken about those things. I pointed out that that was not actually true – only the previous evening I had spoken to Marcia about them. We ended our conversation with Moira saying that I could have the coming weekend as days off, thereby allowing me to travel up north to see Patrick. Keith had generously offered to drive Mother there, so I could travel with them.

Moira could be very generous, and very kind, which made it all the more frustrating when she was awkward or unhelpful.

When I got back to Salisbury, I attended the funeral of Diana's mother-in-law. There I met Pete Day, who had helped me so much as a depressed teenager, for the first time in some years. I told him that I had been in hospital for two months and he gave me his telephone number and told me to contact him if I wanted to.

The following week I went to Carlisle with Mother, my brother Peter and his five-year-old son, Stephen. On the way back from Carlisle, there was a very strange occurrence. We had been travelling for about an hour and I was driving. I was in the righthand lane and I remember signalling and drawing into the middle lane. I then signalled to enter the left hand lane. The next thing I remember was Stephen's voice saying, 'What's happening?' I realised that I was driving on the hard shoulder, because the surface was a pinkish colour whereas the motorway surface was the usual black. I came to a gentle and controlled halt. I put the handbrake on, put the gears into neutral, put my hands into my lap, and said, 'I don't know, Stephen.'

There was a short silence, then Peter asked, 'Are you all right, Vron?'

'I . . . I don't know.' I felt very confused. What was I doing, stopping the car on the hard shoulder? Why had I left the motorway?

'Well, it's all right,' Peter said, wonderfully calming and reassuring. 'Don't worry. Do you want me to drive?'

I nodded, then got slowly out of the car. Peter moved across to the driving seat as I walked around to the passenger side. Mother said nothing, I think she was shocked by what had happened. Peter drove the rest of the way.

I could not understand what had happened, and I had no memory of drawing off the motorway. I had been doing about 70 mph so I must have been breaking for some time. I felt alarmed. What had I done? Why had I done it? Why was there that strange gap in my consciousness? I wondered if I had fallen asleep, yet those occasions I had heard of when people fell asleep at the wheel had resulted in their losing control of the vehicle and having nasty accidents. How could I have maintained such clear control if I had fallen asleep?

On Friday, 20 April 1990, I saw Nick for the first time since my strange driving experience. I told him about it; I felt quite disturbed by it. He admitted that he could not explain it, though he had heard of a similar instance. He said that I should take comfort from the fact that I had maintained control.

We talked about work and Nick noticed that my hands were shaking. He asked me to hold them out in front of me, looked at them shaking before him, then lightly held them by the tips of the fingers, then let them go. He suggested that I reduce the lithium dose to 600 mg as that might help. If the tremble improved, I was to stay at that level; if not, I was to return to the previous level of 800 mg.

This was followed by something of a crisis in the family. Alastair, the son of Jane and John, was admitted to hospital. I went to Surrey, by which time Jane herself had been admitted and was very ill.

I was very anxious when I set off for High Wycombe, for a late shift. Instead of turning off the motorway for High Wycombe, I drove on to Oxford. There I went to Littlemore. I arrived at about eleven in the morning, and walked into Phoenix. None of the nurses saw me when I arrived. I could not bring myself to find anyone, as I felt guilty about being there at all. I went into the low-security A6 corridor and leaned against the windowsill looking out into the courtyard.

I do not know who noticed me there but it was Emma who approached me. 'Veronica,' she said, 'how long have you been here?' I shook my head, if I had wanted to tell her I could not have done. I did not know how long I had been there.

I cannot remember how the ensuing conversation went, though I was not very communicative. Emma said, 'I think you ought to stay with us today.' I said that I was due at work at 13.30. Emma replied, 'I don't think you're fit for work at the moment, are you?' She persuaded me to go into the quad. I gave a glance up, only long enough to identify a safe place to go. This was a chair on its own in the far corner of the room, near the window that I had spent so much time staring out of during my first admission. I sat sideways on the chair so that I had my back to the circle of people that was inevitably there at that time. I sat there, curled up, hiding my face in my hands.

After a little while, someone approached me. She said that she was Anne, an occupational therapist. She was a new member of Phoenix staff whom I did not know.

She stayed and talked to me, got me a cup of tea, and eventually persuaded me to move into the circle. She told me a few times to have a good cry. I felt like saying, what do you mean, a good cry? What will crying do? It just exhausts you and leaves you feeling worse than you did before. She was really very kind but I wished that she would go away.

At some time Emma came back to me. She said that Dr Rose was not in the hospital that day but she had brought Dr Egerton to see me. What was this all about? I was puzzled. I could not understand what was going on; it was all very confusing.

I cannot remember much of what was said in the ensuing interview with Dr Egerton. For some reason Dr Egerton said that I should stay on at Phoenix for a few days. The whole situation was becoming increasingly peculiar. He said something about my being somewhere where I would have people around me at night. Emma added her view. It was very odd.

'How long?' I asked, apparently speaking to the floor.

Dr Egerton said it would probably be just over the weekend, and then they would see how things were. I said that I was all right really, there was nothing wrong with me. Emma said that it was just my saying that that concerned her most. Dr Egerton added his voice to the persuasion saying that I could come and go as I pleased but he felt that I should not be alone at night feeling as I did.

How could I explain the problem? They thought I was ill but I was not really. I was not ill. I was useless and pathetic. I had made a mess of things, again. 'I don't think I *ought* to be here.'

'I think if that is how you feel, we would say that you should stay with us,' Dr Egerton said. I had a problem. I felt vulnerable, threatened, confused and desperately unhappy. I wanted to be, needed to be, somewhere safe, secure. But all this was my fault; all my fault. If I accepted help, it would be an unforgivable weakness. Even if they did not realise it, I knew that I did not deserve help. I wanted help, though. I wanted comfort. I wanted to be looked after.

I was left to think about it. Deborah, Rob and Kevin came up to me individually to encourage me to accept admission. I eventually gave way to the pressure and was admitted in April 1990.

I was given a room on the end of the more secure A7 corridor. It was at the opposite end from that of the first room I had on my first admission. It was basically the same, except that it was a smaller, single room.

There was one good thing about the situation: Nick Rose was out of the hospital. Presumably he would be away until Monday, when I could hopefully leave before he came. He was the last person I wanted to find me there. After all the time, patience and encouragement he had expended on me, the thought of his seeing me there would be too awful. I had my usual depressive thoughts of being inadequate, awfully guilty. I'd made such a mess of things. So many people had done so much for me and look what I had done with it! My sense of failure was centred on Nick Rose because he was the one who had spent most time with me since my discharge.

It was about five or six o'clock, I suppose, when the door opened and someone entered so quickly that it startled me. I was sitting on the side of the bed. It was Nick Rose. If I'd known he were coming, I would have run away.

He smiled and greeted me in his usual courteous manner. He drew up a chair and sat facing me, apologising for 'bursting in on you like this'.

I sat rocking myself, wringing my hands and looking at the floor with the very occasional glance at the person who spoke to me. All the old habits back. I tried to explain myself, justify my presence. I explained what had been happening. Nick listened patiently and sympathetically, commenting that it was not unusual for such things to cause a setback. He said that he would check my drug sheet before he went.

He stood up to go, but before he went he came over and stood by me. He rested his hand on my shoulder and, leaning down to speak quietly, he said that I should stay over the weekend then they would see how I was. He squeezed my shoulder with gentle sympathy. It was as if he was saying, 'I can see how dreadful you are feeling and am sorry to see it. It's all right to be here.' That was what I most needed to be told, it was all right to be there. Now Nick was adding his voice to that of the nurses.

The on-call doctor came to give me the usual physical examination. 'This is a safe place to be, isn't it?' I agreed.

Against expectations, I realised that Nick's visit had helped. I had expected him to say, 'What are you doing here? You shouldn't be here.' Instead I had received a response that was truly compassionate. It is not an easy thing to get through the sense of guilt that is so much a part of depression.

Chapter 13

Lithium levels raised – Attend ward round – Write in
community book – Visit from brother Peter – Discharge

I tried to telephone my cousin Jenny, to tell her of my admission, but she was out so I phoned Peter, who was out, but Sheila answered. I explained that I was in hospital again and asked if she could let Jenny know. Sheila was sympathetic. I telephoned Di but Bryony answered to say that she was at work. The next day she telephoned.

Over the weekend I ate and drank little, did not brush my teeth, wash or change my clothing. For a great majority of the time, I just lay on my bed. Liz, who had been on days during my last admission, was on nights. She would come in and sit back on her heels in front of my bed to speak to me. Her attitude and actions conveyed a real sympathy that could not fail to have an effect. Her action in coming into the room and crossing to my bedside challenged my isolation. She refused to heed my barriers with a gentle disregard for anything other than my need of contact, comfort. She would come into my room each evening, usually asking me to join them if I would like to. This inevitably achieved something and I would usually leave my room after she had gone and sit for a while in the quad.

Monday morning came and I approached Emma and raised the question of my being discharged. She was non-committal and asked if I would mind waiting until she was able to come and talk about it. I went back to my room.

About an hour later Emma came to see me. I sat on the edge of the bed while she moved the chair so that she was facing me. She told me that my case had been discussed in the ward round and the view was that I should stay with them. I was back to all the feelings I had had before the weekend. There was nothing wrong with me, I should not be using their time and energy, there were other people who genuinely needed care. Emma was not deflected by my wish to go. They were not going to prevent me, but Emma made it quite clear that they would be very unhappy if I left. Apart from anything else, I was sufficiently dehydrated to need hospitalisation. It really did seem that she believed I should stay, that I needed to be there, that I was ill and needed to be in hospital. In the end, I gave in and agreed to stay.

Emma was right about my dehydration. By Monday afternoon I had a coarse tremor, the floor had developed a disconcerting habit of moving about, I had loose bowel movements despite having eaten practically nothing – I should have been constipated – and I had increasing nausea. I spoke to Linda, who said she would speak to the doctors. I approached her later and she was surprised that no one had seen me.

Ultimately, no one did come. I did not like to make a fuss since I was probably simply being over-anxious. I increased my fluid intake from Monday evening but I did not have blood taken for levels until Thursday morning. The lithium must have been at its highest over Sunday evening/Monday morning. The level on Thursday would certainly have been lower, yet it was still 0.93 mmol/l, higher than it had ever been.

On Tuesday I went into the nursing office where Tim was on his own. I asked if I would be disturbing him if I went in and he said I would not, he was just getting some off-duty done. I went in and sat down. I made some comments, which he found difficult to hear. He eventually said that either I would have to look up or he would have to get nearer. He put the off-duty down and came to sit by me. I talked about the frustrations I was suffering.

Tim listened sympathetically. Eventually, though, he interrupted and said that what really needed attention immediately were my basic needs – my priority, right then, should be to get some food and fluids inside me. 'Here,' he said, 'why don't you have a fluid chart, you can keep it yourself, you know how much fluid you should be drinking in this weather.'

On Wednesday morning there was a knock on the door. I opened it to a dark-haired young man whose identity I was initially unsure of. He politely asked if I would mind coming into the ward round with him. I realised that this doctor was Michael Egerton. I had not looked at him when I met him before.

I was rather amazed at the request for me to go into the ward round. I had not been asked during my previous admissions. All I knew about going to a ward round was from being present at a few conversations when it was discussed. During my first admission, I heard one of the other patients talk about being asked to attend the ward round. She sounded resentful and cynical, suggesting that all those present had been enjoying her discomfiture. She implied that all they invited a patient in for was their own entertainment. I found this difficult to believe, partly because the patient concerned seemed to have an attitude that was generally bitter and cynical. Of course, I know rather more than most about what goes on when doctors and nurses get together to discuss patients, and therefore I was prepared to take their good faith on trust. It had never occurred to me that I would be invited to a ward round.

I was surprised as Michael Egerton led me through the quad and on past the central office. Ward rounds had always been held in the blue room previously. As Dr Egerton held the door open and I walked in, I glanced up very briefly. Nick Rose stood up and said, 'Hello Veronica, come and sit by me.'

I sat down and fixed my eyes on the floor. Nick leaned towards me and spoke quietly. He told me that Dr Egerton, whom I knew, was seated on the other side of me, and Rob was there. He also told me that there were some medical students present. He said that he thought I would know the other people there. This was both helpful and reassuring as, on entry, I had very much felt that the room was full of strangers.

He asked a few introductory questions. I commented that I seemed to have become all shaky and jumpy again. He responded in sympathetic agreement. He went on to explain that they wondered what I thought should happen next. I paused, glanced at him, then said that I was next due at work a week on Friday.

'And you'd like to aim at getting back to work then?' Nick asked. I nodded. 'Yes,' he said, 'I think it would be reasonable.' When my idea of what I should be doing coincided with that of the Phoenix staff, it suggested that my view of the situation at last bore some relation to reality. The outcome of my conversation with Nick Rose was that I should aim to go home before or after the weekend, as I thought best. He finished by asking if there were any questions that I would like to ask. This was how he always ended discussions with me when I was in such a state – when more myself I could be relied on to put forward whatever questions I wished to. I said that I had no questions.

Nick got to his feet as I rose to leave, and thanked me for coming. Michael Egerton went out of the room with me. He also thanked me for coming and said that I had done very well. He asked me if I would like him to walk me back to the room, but I declined. Dr Egerton was sensitive in his approach and very polite. I had got on with Steve Johnson reasonably well but I could not imagine him taking such an approach. When you feel nervous and vulnerable, you need that sort of careful reassurance without which you would normally cope quite well.

By the time of my last few days on the ward, I really began to come out of myself. I was still not sleeping well, tending to wake early and to stay awake. I made use of this, however, by getting up and leaving my room. I then had the hour before the arrival of the day staff and breakfast at eight o'clock to sit and talk to the nurses. I had discovered how useful it could be to be up and about early. I did wonder why I had not discovered it sooner. Early one morning I had quite a long chat with Rob. Since I was the only patient up, he was able to give me his undivided attention.

I was much more forthcoming during the last two community meetings I attended during that admission than I had ever been before. Jonathon, a staff nurse new to the ward, Martin and I had quite a conversation about what had and had not been helpful for nurses to do for me while I had been isolating myself. I said that there were two people who had particularly helped me during the first stages of that admission – Nick Rose and Liz, who was on nights. From each of those persons I got a sense of compassion, physical and emotional, that prompted them to approach me. The message I received, that 'it is all right to be here', was very much needed by me. I spoke of this, and other things that had been helpful to me. Jonathon thanked me after the meeting, for what I had said, as he had found it very useful.

During the time I was in Phoenix, the favourite game of both staff and patients was Scrabble. I was playing with Martin one evening and he put down 'ai' and, when I challenged it, he managed to convince me that it was a legitimate word – a three-toed sloth, apparently. We speculated on the possibility that three toes were insufficient to keep the sloth on the tree and that *ai!* was the cry it made as it fell off the branch.

One evening I was in the nursing office when Karen was trying to persuade Joe, a young teenage patient who had been in hospital a long time but was then due for discharge, that it would be a good idea to get out of bed before lunchtime. Karen was interrupted by the arrival of Wayne, who announced that he would cut the fingers off whoever had stolen his sweets, then left.

Karen had been trying to encourage Joe to write something in the diary for that day but, since he showed no sign of doing so, I picked up the book. I had never written anything in the diary. I wrote:

> I am writing this since Joe, although not having been in his usual state of rigor mortis during daylight hours, has apparently forgotten how to write. Wayne has threatened to cut the fingers off the person who stole his sweeties, so whoever it was had better eat them while he still has the fingers to get them out of the bag. I had better not write any more in case those mentioned object. Ai would then be a three-toed sloth, i.e. a combination of Joe and whoever stole Wayne's sweeties.

Karen read it and laughed. Later that evening Joe was in the office trying to find the diary to find out what I had written about him, but Linda had hidden it. The next morning Karen said to me, 'You're quite a wit, aren't you? I was chuckling all the way home last night.'

My first reaction on being told that I could go either before or after the weekend was to say that I would go on Friday. Peter had telephoned at the beginning of the week to say that he and Sheila would be happy to have me at any time.

On the afternoon of the Thursday, Emma came to my room to tell me that Peter was there to visit. I was surprised, as I had not been expecting him. After I greeted Peter with a hug I went into the nursing office to tell Emma that Peter and I would be going out for a while. 'You didn't tell me that you had a good-looking brother like that,' she said.

We went down to Sandford Lock and sat by the river. Peter was glad to see how I was as he had been expecting me to be as I had been during my first admission.

Chapter 14

Visits from family – Role of friends – Sidney stays – Locked
wards – Friends – Hospital facilities – Other professionals

Geographically, my nearest relative was my cousin, Jennifer. Our
mothers were sisters – Jenny came from Cornwall where she had
grown up on the farm that I so much loved to visit. I still visit the
farm where Jenny's brother Peter and sister-in-law Sharon now live,
whenever I can, which is not as often as I would like. Jenny lives in
Thame, about fifteen miles away from Oxford on the same side as
Littleworth and Wheatley, where I came to live. Jenny has always
been very supportive and helpful to me in any way she can. She was
one of my more frequent visitors.

Of course, one of my problems was that my family was rather
scattered and none of them lived in Oxford. Keith and Clare lived
in Arborfield, near Reading, but they both worked full time and
had two young children to bring up. Eleanor, in Chalfont-St-Giles,
was in much the same position. When I was well, I greatly enjoyed
looking after the children. I have seventeen nieces and nephews and
it has been lovely watching them each grow up. Although we are a
large family, we get together whenever we can. My fortieth birthday was celebrated with a party in the house where Jane and John

then lived in Surrey. They hired a gazebo from the scouts and it was a lovely mild evening so we sat outside talking until we decided that it was too late to be disturbing the neighbours. All my brothers and sisters and in-laws were there with their children. Patrick and Kathleen came all the way from Carlisle, Kathy and her husband from Derbyshire, and Katherine and Nicholas from Nailsea. My friend Cathy, with whom I did the neonatal course, travelled from Thame, as did Jenny and her daughter.

Things were much easier when I was out of hospital, especially those times when I was able to drive and so visit people. When I was an inpatient, things were rather more problematic. Most people had to travel – and to travel some distance – in order to visit. This meant that some weeks went by when I was not visited by any of my family. During the first years of my illness, they had young families as well as the problems of travelling long distances, and only having the weekends to do things at home. However, they all managed to visit on occasion. I especially liked to see the children.

Jane, who lived in Surrey at the time, and Diana in Salisbury, were my most consistent visitors, and remained so. They would also bring my mother or my father. Mother already had experience of the difficulties of getting from Salisbury to Oxford on public transport, from when she first came. She would bring her Cairn terrier, Sidney, who became quite a celebrity on the ward. I always enjoyed seeing him. If I was able to, I would go out with Jane or Diana. We would usually go for a pub lunch. There was a village near Littlemore with a large green in the middle. Jane, Mother and I went to the pub on the green for lunch. I always remember that day as Jane took a photograph of Mother and me sitting on the bench on the green, with me holding Sidney by the lead.

On one occasion when Nick insisted that I should be admitted, I was looking after Sidney for Mother. No one could come to collect him for three days, so I said that I couldn't go into hospital. Sandra Young, who was the senior nurse at Phoenix as well as my named nurse, said, 'Well, bring Sidney.' So Sid came with me and slept under the bed. Elaine, the SHO, became very fond of Sidney, who always enjoyed her making a fuss of him when she came to my room. One day she came to invite me to attend the ward round. I was shutting Sid in behind me when she said, 'Oh, aren't you bringing Sidney? I told them all about him and they want to meet him,' so Sid came too.

When I was last admitted, in June 2007, I was in Nick Rose's newly built ward at the Warneford. My friend Mia was looking after my own little dog, Millie. She brought her to visit me but they wouldn't allow her on the ward. Somewhat reluctantly, they allowed Mia to take her into the garden – surrounded by a tall fence with newly planted bushes all around. There was a gate directly into the garden, which was normally kept locked, and Millie was allowed through there so I could see her in the garden. I got the impression that they were not particularly happy even with that.

Most of the time I was in Phoenix, except for the very last admissions, the ward was unlocked. However, they have now started to keep the doors of the ward locked. I had always thought that the unlocking of the wards was regarded as a great advance in psychiatry, yet here they were taking an apparently retrograde step. Since 2007, this policy has become adopted throughout the Warneford and Littlemore hospitals. There has also been a change in the use of the wards, with Phoenix becoming a rehabilitation ward (although I hear that it has since been declared an acute ward again, by the ward manager). Nick's ward was changed to a new ward at the Warneford, where all the acute wards now are, called Allen ward. This ward is also locked. Although it has a small garden, it is surrounded by a rather forbiddingly high fence. It makes it feel like a secure ward even if it is not supposed to be, and I find this unpleasant. I assumed that the fact that keys are no longer needed by staff – all they need is a small swipe card – was one of the main reasons for locking the wards. Keeping control of the patients is no longer problematic.

Yesterday I met one of the ward managers, whom I know, and she told me that the ostensible reason for locking wards was to keep people out – locals had found that Phoenix and Ashurst were nice places to play snooker free of charge. I expressed some dubiety about this, pointing out that it could be easy enough to monitor more closely who was coming in without it being necessary to lock the doors. It seems to be rather too convenient that this resulted in locking in the patients and only allowing out those who had permission. The ward manager agreed with me, saying that they had been against it.

I spoke to Tim, my community psychiatric nurse, about it. He admitted that the ward he had worked on in London had been locked, though he agreed with me that there was a large element of controlling patients in the locked doors policy. I commented that when I had been on a psychiatric ward at the Whittingdon Hospital, in London, the door had been open but there was always a nurse who sat there to prevent any patient from leaving who was not allowed to do so. I admitted that it must have been a rather boring job, but expressed the belief that a rota with a frequent change of door attendant could surely be devised. Personally, I feel that the present political concerns about psychiatric patients absconding, and the fears of the public – largely exaggerated – are being pandered to instead of disproved by the facts of the situation. (For it has recently been said that you are more likely to win the lottery than be killed by a mental patient.) I am sure there is a political element to this.

I did, of course, have many friends around Oxford and in Wheatley. Katherine and Nicholas were regular visitors and I missed them very much when they moved to Nailsea. Subsequently, they had to move again, to Saffron Walden near Cambridge. This was worse, if anything; at least when they were in Nailsea they were conveniently close to Peter and Sheila in Yate, near Bristol, so when I went to stay with them I could visit Katherine and Nicholas.

I attended a church house group each Monday evening. My friends there were very supportive. When I was allowed home for the day, or longer, Jennifer was very good at arranging for herself or someone else to pick me up from the hospital and take me home, or back to Littlemore. Nona was the other person Jennifer usually enrolled to be my chauffeur if she herself was unavailable. I also attend a morning prayer breakfast at half-past seven on a Thursday at the United Reformed Church. I was one of six stalwarts who were almost always there. This group was very supportive, too. Wendy used the delay mechanism on her camera to take a photograph of all of them and they made it into a card for me and sent it to Phoenix.

During most of the time things were at their worst, John Fuller was the vicar at St Mary's. He would come to visit me and always offered his full support. Since then he and his wife, Gill, have moved down to Shaftesbury, as John has retired. That is reasonably near Salisbury, so I can go to see them when I am there; it is nice to keep in touch with them.

When I was able to, it was nice to go out with visitors. A pub lunch was the favourite, but it was often pleasant just to go back to the flat. Once I had Millie (she was usually looked after by Jenny in Thame) when I was in hospital. I always used to love Millie's visits and she would get very excited when she saw me.

I found that being confined to the ward was very difficult. It felt as if I were imprisoned, much as the nurses who cared for me would hate the analogy. It is a peculiar and unpleasant experience. Policemen occasionally returned me to the hospital. They were always pleasant to me. I knew that they were returning me under their right to take me to a 'place of safety'. But as a policeman who found me in my car said, 'I am giving you no choice.' The police always contacted Phoenix if they had found me not as a result of the nurses having reported me missing. If Phoenix staff told them that I was sectionable, they had the right to return me – with no choice. It is not an experience a law-abiding citizen normally has. I remember when I was a teenager, going for a long walk along a country road and sitting on the grass verge as dusk came. A police car drew up. The policeman questioned me and, having established that I was over sixteen, drove away leaving me where I was. They had no cause to do otherwise. Finding out that I was a sectionable psychiatric patient was another matter. Having your freedom very much restricted is a peculiar experience. Fortunately, the ward would make every effort to allow me out with my visitors, and even if it was only a walk around the grounds, it would be very enjoyable, especially if I otherwise had to wait for a nurse to escort me.

When I was very disturbed, I would often behave impulsively – most often in the form of trying to leave the ward, causing the nurses to have to bring me back if I succeeded. I would be obsessed with the idea of going home. On one occasion I actually managed to get home. I was taking tablets out of their foil packages when I knocked a box over and foil packs went all over the floor. At that moment there was a loud knock on the door. I ignored it initially, but there was another loud knock. I opened it to find a policeman on my doorstep. He was talking to my neighbour, who was saying that I might be working. She went inside when I opened the door. The policeman turned his attention to me. 'Veronica,' he said, inviting himself in. 'It is Veronica, isn't it? Shall we have a chat?' He saw the tablets on the floor and asked me why they were there. I said I had knocked them accidentally. At some time he picked them up and put them into their boxes. He asked me if I wanted him to take me back to Littlemore, but I shook my head.

He used my telephone to talk to someone at the hospital. I gathered from the conversation that some nurses were coming to return me to the ward. He told them that I had tablets, but had not taken any and said he would stay with me until they came. 'Did you get that?' he asked me when he came off the telephone. I nodded.

He sat at the table and picked up a book, *Wellington's Peninsular Victories*, that I had just finished reading. He remarked that it was unusual material for a woman and said that it was a period he was interested in. He pulled a biography of Wellington from the pile and said that he had just been given that book for his birthday. He looked around my bookshelves and commented, 'You're a heavy reader, a very heavy reader.'

The policeman was looking out of the window when he commented that a car was approaching slowly. Apparently it went past and then returned. He remarked that they must be looking for somewhere to park.

One nurse, whom I did not recognise, came up and the policeman let him in. He introduced himself. It was, however, mainly the policeman who persuaded me to go with him.

The next day three nurses returned me to the ward after I had left once again, but not gone very far. Later that day a nurse was in my room and I told her that I wanted to cut my throat or my wrists. She said that I might not do it properly but I pointed out that I knew where my arteries were. She was very concerned about this, as violent plans are often most serious. She eventually told me that if I continued like that she would have to get a doctor who would section me.

The day after, I was sitting on the low shelf out in the corridor when a nurse came up and asked me to come to see Dr Lane, but I shook my head. She tried, without success, to persuade me. The doctor then came forward, asked me to come to talk with her and gently held my hand while leading me to one of the interview rooms.

The doctor was very gentle and spoke carefully to me. She asked me the usual questions and I told her what I had told the nurse, that I would cut my throat. After a while she got up and left the room. I sat alone for a while then got up and left the room. I walked out of the main door. There was a bus at the stop but it left straight away. I wandered towards the hospital exit, then became aware of someone walking towards me. It was Dr Lane and a nurse. I commented that I had missed the bus. They persuaded me to return to the interview room. The doctor had been telephoning Nick. She told me that they were very worried about me so I would have one nurse assigned to me, which, she said, could be nice because I would always have a nurse with me. The last time this was a possibility Nick had asked the nurses to look in on me every five minutes, as close observation was so invasive. It was not to be.

Things had changed since I had been in the old hospital over the road. Then you were left alone in your room with the occasional check. Now the nurse had to have you continuously in sight. When I went into my room and lay on the bed, the door would be left open; the nurse would sit on a chair in the doorway. If I wanted to go to the toilet, a female nurse would accompany me into the ladies and I could only push the door to close it, never lock it. I stayed on these observations for the weekend and beyond.

Nick came to see me with two medical students. I told him that I felt better and he commented that he could have a conversation with me, but that in contrast when things were bad, he could hardly get a word out of me. It had been like that before the weekend. He said that I could go on to fifteen-minute observations and commented that the trifluorperazine I had been receiving to help my thoughts and tendency to act impulsively had been effective. The dose had been quickly increased but now that I was obviously improving, it was being slowly brought down.

My level of freedom was always increased as I improved. There were places within the hospital that I could go to on my own, if I were allowed. It may not sound very important, but I could go to the hospital hairdresser. It was actually quite an enhancement to your morale to have your hair cut and made decent, especially after a period of self-neglect. When I had gone for some weeks not being able to leave the ward, it was nice to go and have my hair done. Originally it was free for patients, but a charge was introduced, which was then put up a few times. However, it remains very good value – a good deal cheaper than having Millie's coat cut! – and I have always used it as an outpatient.

There was a gym in the old Phoenix, that was installed while I was there. When I was confined to the hospital, it was good to get some exercise. The gym was moved to the new hospital and I tried to get to it twice a week. It has the advantage of being staffed by qualified physiotherapists and is free to use. At one time there was a senior physiotherapist who was trained in reflexology, and I used to go for a very relaxing session once a week. I do not know how much it would have cost in a commercial setting, but I was lucky to have those sessions. Unfortunately that physiotherapist left the hospital and there was no one to take over from her in that capacity.

One tends to think of hospitals as being staffed by doctors and the nurses, but there were so many other professionals involved with my care: the housekeepers, who kept the hospital clean – very successfully – and served meals; psychotherapists; physiotherapists; occupational therapists; Anne, the hairdresser; and many other people. It is quite surprising who can become involved in care in a modern hospital.

Chapter 15

My sister Diana talks to Nick Rose – Problems at work with
Marcia – Moira sees me on return from her long absence,
extremely critical – I see personnel officer – Criticisms in
writing – Admission to Phoenix – Show Tim critical letter

On leaving Littlemore, I stayed with Peter and Sheila for a few days then returned to Salisbury. On 15 May 1990, I drove to Oxford with Diana. We had an appointment to see Nick Rose together. After a pub lunch, we went to Littlemore. Di had suggested that it might help if he saw her with me. When I put this to him he said that he would be quite happy to see Diana if I thought it would be useful. He proved quite happy to meet with anyone who I asked him to see. When we arrived in his secretary's office, Nick was making himself a coffee; he offered us one, which Diana accepted.

Diana made some interesting comments about me as a child. She said that I was between Patrick, who was a very lively and attractive child, always a favourite with Mother, and Clare who was very determined and demanding of Mother's attention. She described me as 'a very affectionate child'. This surprised me – I had never been aware of myself as an affectionate child. I repeated Di's comment to Jane and she agreed, adding that I was also a very happy child. This I knew was true. In photographs of me as a child, I am always laughing or smiling, in contrast to Clare, who always had a rather grim and determined expression, looking serious. I also knew, however, that I was a very quiet child, undemanding of attention – which did not mean that I did not want attention.

Nick asked Diana to judge how far I was like my normal self, on a percentage scale with 100% being normal for me. Di said I was certainly beyond halfway, but still had a long way to go. I put the same question to Peter, who replied, 'No more than 50% to 55%,' which I suppose accorded with what Diana said.

As we went back to the car, Diana remarked of Nick Rose 'He's nice, isn't he? I can imagine him with his children.' That, coming from Diana for whom her children were the most important thing in her life, was certainly a compliment.

I went back to work on an early shift on Friday, 11 May, as planned. The following Wednesday I went to see Reverend Andrew Wilson, the hospital's non-medical advisor, for a general chat and to let him know how I was getting on. I mentioned that I was writing an article with a view towards possible publication. Andrew thought that this was a positive sign. Before I went, he gave me the name of another priest who would be able to fulfil the role of non-medical advisor, and let me have his number. I was surprised at this, though it was explained the next time I saw Andrew. It was at work, as he had come on to the unit to see the parents of one of our babies. He came to speak to me before he left. He said that he would be going in two weeks. I asked him where he was going and he told me that he was leaving All Saints to go to Cambridge. He was surprised that I did not know.

I next saw him just before he left – he and his family were getting into the car. I handed him a card and a letter. I had had to think hard over the letter, it was not easy to express how important his help had been to me, or how grateful I was to him. Reverend Andrew Wilson was, in every sense, a godly man.

I started full-time work again in the first week of July 1990. This was not out of choice but because I had used up a lot of annual leave and needed to keep some for holidays later in the year. I was not looking forward to a full week's work, sensing that it would be a strain, not only in regard to the hours worked but also because of the reduction in hours away from work to recover. The off-duty was so written that I had six consecutive days on, including four early shifts together. I was afraid that I would find it too tiring, but also had a sense of guilt about having such a negative attitude – things were bound to go wrong if I expected them to. The situation was not helped when someone asked me how I was, remarking that I looked dreadfully tired.

I had left SCBU the previous July with the feeling that morale among the staff was very low. Talking to Dianne one day I remarked on how discouraging it was to come back and find that things were as bad as ever. 'It's worse,' was her immediate retort. I received the same response from another member of staff. I felt better for knowing that I was not the only one who thought that there were problems on SCBU.

I had been working in the hot nursery for a few weeks before I took on the care of intensive care babies. I was initially given the care of a ventilated baby and one ready for transference to an incubator, when Marcia, who was in charge, asked Rose to take care of them. Rose, not a specialist qualified nurse, felt that she could not take on the responsibility. I was washing my hands in the nearby sink and said that I would be happy to have the babies. Marcia asked if I thought I could cope and I assured her that I could. I would not have offered otherwise. I quite enjoyed caring for a ventilated baby again. That day Marcia was quite busy and let me get on with things. It was not so busy the next day, however, and she started to watch over me, even reminding me to keep up with my observations, one of the most fundamental tasks. I would probably not normally have reacted with such annoyance, but then Marcia would not normally watch over me. It seemed to me that she simply did not trust me.

One morning I left report early in order to relieve Maggie, the night charge nurse, from care of a ventilated baby, and I voiced my frustration. Maggie laughed and said that I should come on to nights – she would allocate a ventilated baby to me and let me get on with it. I commented on the fact that, the previous July no one had expressed any concern about my competence, or found it necessary to watch over me even when I was on the verge of a total collapse. No one had even noticed. Maggie responded a little indignantly to that, saying that they had noticed. I was tempted to ask why no one had done anything about it, but decided not to.

The third day I was on an early. Marcia asked Steph, a specialist enrolled nurse, to take the ventilated baby. I felt very fed-up and was, I suspect, somewhat irritable. Marcia clearly showed that she did not trust me with a sick child. Quite honestly I felt insulted, particularly since Marcia was not the most clinically brilliant of nurses on the unit. I felt a bit mean, thinking like that. I liked Marcia personally, she was a very genuine person, kind and caring – but she had no right to watch over me. The truth was that I was genuinely demoralised and morale among the unit staff was not high. I found full-time work demanding, particularly when being at work was draining my confidence. I felt untrusted, unappreciated and belittled. I was tired, disillusioned and losing faith in myself. Just when I most needed encouragement, I was faced with criticism and lack of trust. I could not build up my confidence when faced with distrust.

During the course of a morning I noticed that there was a fault on a cardiac monitor. The baby attached to that monitor was being cared for by Marcia. In addition, Marcia was the nurse in charge. I decided that it would be better for me to tell Marcia about the fault rather than to do anything myself, which might have been construed as interfering. I pointed out the fault, which probably arose from someone's having set the parameters wrongly. I moved away to do something else when Marcia said, 'You know, Veronica, when you see something wrong you should put it right.' Considering the mood I was in, that comment was best greeted with silence. I told myself to say nothing, but the temptation was too much. I could not disguise my irritation. 'I am trying to, Marcia,' I said through clenched teeth. I remembered Moira's words to me after the grading appeal – 'I know who I can rely on to notice things and put them right.' Marcia's remark was grossly unjust when addressed to me. In this particular instance I had failed to put things right myself because I did not want to be seen as interfering by doing it for her. It seemed that I could not do right for doing wrong.

Marcia said she wanted a word with me in the office. That was all I needed.

I cannot remember most of what Marcia said, except that it was very damning of me. She said that it was my attitude that really concerned her. She was trying to be nice – if someone is taking a hostile stance it is easy for you to steel yourself against it, but when they are obviously making an effort to be nice it is more problematic. I stood, propping myself against a pile of chairs and the tears began to fall. Marcia was obviously affected by my distress. 'Listen, love,' she said, 'I know you've been demoralised lately.'

'Marcia, I've been demoralised for the last two years!'

Marcia left me alone in the office to recover. She came in later and suggested that I go and have a coffee. I ended up in the staff cloakroom trying, not very successfully, to stop crying. Marcia came and suggested I do a split-shift – going home and coming back later. This proved to be the incentive I needed. I took a deep breath and told Marcia that I was all right. I splashed my face with water, dried it, then went back to the nursery.

Steph joined me in the sitting room at lunchtime. She asked me what was wrong, I looked so unhappy. I explained as well as I could.

Steph was sympathetic and above all, positive, in response. 'You're as good as any of them,' she stated.

I said that I was no longer sure if I could do my own job. 'Yes, you can,' Steph answered, very forthrightly. 'Don't you let them say you can't.' If it were not for Steph, I do not think that I could have got through to the end of the shift.

Marcia had no comprehension of demoralisation as I knew it – feeling totally unappreciated and unvalued. Steph understood what I was saying.

When I went to Littlemore and saw Nick Rose and told him something of what had happened at work. I expressed my frustration at not being trusted. I described what had happened between Marcia and me but said that I had begun to feel better since then (almost a week ago). However, he felt sufficiently happy with my progress to reduce the amitriptyline dose to 150 mg. Nick told me that he would be away for much of August and would not see me until September.

I went down to my cousin's farm in Cornwall before returning to work. When I went on duty, Moira was in the office. I asked her how she was because she had been off sick for a month, coming back just after I went away on annual leave. We exchanged the usual pleasantries, then Moira said she wanted to see me later. This did not surprise me, though the content of the interview did. I was not at all prepared for the extreme nature of her criticism. I was stunned. Perhaps I should not have been surprised, as there was nothing new about it after what had happened over the gradings. I should have had an idea of what to expect. I got the impression that Moira was deliberately taking advantage of what she perceived as my vulnerability. I also felt that she had come back from sick leave and saw an opportunity to launch an attack and was not going to let it pass. Given my annual leave and her sick leave, she had not seen me at work for at least six weeks.

She said a lot of things, some of which I tried to answer, though I soon gave that up. It seemed to me that she did not intend to recognise that I had a right to have my view heard. She was not going to entertain the idea that I had a valid viewpoint.

One of the comments she made in the first few minutes was, 'Nick's not back until the 20th and I can't wait until then.' Obviously she had telephoned Littlemore to talk to Nick Rose without my permission or knowledge, which was a clear breach of confidentiality as she must well have known. I felt annoyed at this typically high-handed action of Moira's. She clearly believed that he would have spoken to her, without consulting me, and that he would be sympathetic to her viewpoint. In fact, there was no way he would have spoken to her about me without my express permission.

Moira implied that all or most of my colleagues were offended by my attitude and manner. I suggested that it would be better if individuals would approach me personally. Moira's response was, 'They're afraid that they might upset you.' I answered the point saying that I was a good deal more upset to have everything thrown at me at once. Moira repeated her previous answer, adding, 'After all, you have had a *mental* illness.' Well, you could not trust these mental cases; upset them and you never know what they would do. This was my first experience of blatant prejudice against those with psychiatric histories. Moira did not herself seem to be affected by the serious risk inherent in criticising the insane.

During the course of Moira's ensuing lecture she said that she had taken advice from personnel, and suggested that I see the personnel officer myself. I agreed, with some cynicism; given Moira's attitude, I could not see anything that would improve the situation.

Moira did make comments about my 'undermining colleagues in their use of technical equipment'. I deduced, from what she said, that she was referring to the incident with Marcia over the cardiac monitor. To the comment implying that I avoided putting things right, to which I quite justifiably objected, I replied, 'There is no one who has the right to put that criticism to me.' I looked straight at Moira – she looked away without answering my point. Frustrating as always, I could never call her to account; if she did not like what I said, she simply ignored it.

The interview went in a way that had become familiar to me. Moira was heavily critical of me, while refusing to allow me to have a fair say by ignoring or avoiding my points in my own defence. It made me feel increasingly frustrated, angry and hopeless. What chance had I got of a fair hearing? What had I done to deserve this vilifying attack? I began to feel an immense sense of futility. What was the point of trying at all? I gave up trying to argue my case and sat back and listened with increasing cynicism.

Before I left, Moira telephoned and made an appointment to see the personnel officer on 9 August 1990 – my birthday. Her last comment was that personnel had told her to put everything in writing – and so to give me all the evidence I needed. It proved what I had been saying about her behaviour. When I saw the woman from personnel, I noticed that she did not advise me to put everything in writing – presumably my view was not as important.

My late shift was followed by two earlies – I had to push myself to work, for I felt like sitting down and giving up altogether.

On the Thursday I saw the personnel officer. She was very nice but didn't inspire me with confidence. She told me how concerned Sister Campbell obviously was for me. That was suitably impressed upon me. I tried a test question, pointing out that Moira had telephoned Nick Rose without my knowledge or permission. She said that I did not know that she had telephoned to actually talk to him – perhaps she wanted to find out if I could see him. 'Sister Campbell knows quite well that all I need do if I want to see Dr Rose is to telephone his secretary.' She had no answer for that – given that she had no intention of actually admitting the simple fact that it was a breach of confidentiality. Even when I made a clear statement to the fact, she would not concede.

I asked whether our conversation was in confidence. I would have had more faith in her if she had given me a straight 'no' in reply, but she just avoided the question and went on to something else. Our meeting ended with her telling me that she was there for me as well – who did she think she was fooling?

That afternoon I was in the clinical room when Marcia handed me a brown envelope with a typed address to 'Staff Nurse V Burton, SCBU'. Opening it, I discovered that this was what Moira meant by putting it in writing. I did not read it then.

At home, alone, I had a look at the paper the envelope contained. It was very formal and official. It purported to be an 'Advice and Counselling Session'. Not my idea of counselling. I felt there was a deliberate attempt to intimidate me. I did not read the whole thing then – it was weeks before I was able to do that. What was in the envelope was not so much critical as vitriolic. Months later, when I remarked to Kathleen that I did not think Moira was being malicious (wishful thinking on my part), Kath answered, 'There's definitely malice in that.' I had never been the recipient of such criticism. I was appalled and dismayed.

Among other things, it referred to 'Complaints from two mothers . . . complaints from a doctor.' I was highly dubious of these. Where was the evidence? I thought. If official complaints were being made, then written statements should have been taken. So it went on [my addition in brackets]:

rudeness and aggression to a sister . . .

Intolerance of many colleagues' about their confidence with machinery, thus undermining their confidence and creating an unpleasant atmosphere within the nursery area . . . mood swings . . . lack of insight . . .

I [Moira] have to consider the morale of the parents and

the whole nursing and medical staff . . . need to change . . .
attitude to parents . . . attitude to all your colleagues . . .

She even said I was 'aware' in the same paragraph as she said I
'lacked total insight'.

I read the letter in small excerpts, when I felt strong enough.
I was devastated. I thought of telephoning Phoenix that first night
I received it, for someone to talk to, but decided against it – they
might think that there was something wrong with me.

The interview with Vivienne the next day was decidedly unpro-
ductive. I could not speak and could not explain, apart from to say it
was something at work. At the end, Vivienne asked if I would mind
if she talked to Nick Rose. I said I did not. Vivienne then reminded
me that I could telephone Phoenix at any time.

That afternoon I went to Witney to see Katherine. She sat on the
floor, feeding the baby in his bouncer with one hand and the other
on mine, and listened to me. She had obviously realised that something was wrong though I, as usual, was unaware of how abnormal
my behaviour was. I told her about Moira's letter. Putting both her
hands in mine she said that she and Nick would do anything they
could to help, it did not matter how often I needed their help. They
would always be there because they loved me, they would always be
there whenever I needed them. I had told her that I was afraid that
people would run out of patience with me. She knew about those
fears, and was doing all she could to allay them, to reassure me. It
was such a lovely and loving thing to say – and they were always
there for me, through all the years my depression affected me.

I asked Katherine what I should do. She suggested that I telephone Phoenix as they had always been so good before. I could
not say yes or no. She held her hands in mine again, said that she
thought we ought to pray, then phone Phoenix.

Katherine telephoned, then took me to Littlemore. Rob saw me
with her. He asked the usual questions. Then he said, 'Are you eating – or more important, drinking?' This was something Katherine
was worried about – I had had no more than a few sips of the drinks
she had given me.

Rob said he thought that I ought to see the duty doctor. He told
me that she was Patricia Hart, who had worked alongside Steve the
year before, so I knew her.

Patricia was as I remembered her, quite forthright in her approach.
She directed some of her questions to Katherine. 'What made you
feel that Veronica is not herself?'

Katherine said that I spoke very quietly, I did not look at her, and
I seemed unable to make even the most simple decisions.

Patricia asked me to go through what I had done that day. When I admitted that I had got a prescription she asked me if I had the drugs. They took them from me. Patricia suggested that I should be admitted but I adamantly refused. In the end it was decided that I should go back with Katherine, who would bring me in the next morning to spend the day at Phoenix. Patricia said she would prescribe me 100 mg of chlorpromazine, as I really needed to sleep.

Saturday I was in the ward office when Patricia came in and asked how I was. 'All right,' I replied.

'You don't look it!' she retorted categorically.

I sat on the bench in the courtyard. Patricia came out with the ward's new registrar, whom she introduced as Angela. She remarked, as Patricia had the night before, that Nick Rose had not made arrangements to see me until September and had reduced my medication. He must have thought that I was doing well. She asked me what had happened to change that. I said that I had had problems with my senior nurse, but nothing else. Once again they suggested admission and I refused. The registrar asked me what I had planned to do that weekend. I said that I was going to my sister's in Reading. I was told not to drive and that I should ask Clare to come and get me. I thought it was too far and it would make more sense to stay at Witney. Angela was not keen on this – she asked me how my friend's husband felt. He was as supportive as Katherine, I told her, quite truthfully. I was frustrated.

Angela said she was sure that Clare would come and get me, adding that depressed people often underestimated how much people were prepared to help. I felt that was beside the point.

I was left to think about it before taking it upon myself to telephone Katherine and ask her to come and get me.

My old fear, ECT, had been raised that afternoon. I could not believe there was any need for that but was told that if I was not better by Monday, then they would consider it. With Nick Rose away, this was an ominous development.

Mike came out to talk to me like he had promised. I told him that the problem was at work. He said that I should concern myself with more immediate problems – by Monday, the earth might have opened and swallowed Wycombe SCBU. I then said I did not want to talk about ECT and he accepted that. He had sympathised before, so I trusted him to be my advocate.

On Monday morning I saw the registrar and Sylvia, a nurse who was new to me – she had just returned from a course. Angela thought that I was no better and decided I should be admitted. I was more adamant then ever in my refusal. The registrar and Sylvia were insistent. I even surprised myself in my determination not to go into hospital. Angela had to go, leaving Sylvia to keep up the pressure. I remember her saying, 'Veronica, I don't think you'd recognise me if you met me in the street, you have not looked at me once.' She went on, 'You know we could put you on a section, but we're not going to do that . . .'

I was not sure what the purpose of that remark was, though I thought it was somewhat disingenuous.

I was admitted to Phoenix again on 13 August 1990. Initially I told no one about the letter until Tim was in my room one day, using his height at my request to close my window, high up by the ceiling as it was. Before he went I handed him the letter, and at some pretext left the room while he read it.

When I came back he looked at me and said, 'You know, you have got to answer this.' He then asked if he could tell Nick about it, since he was back by then, and I said yes.

Later I went to Tim and gave him a piece of paper. He started to read, with a slight, puzzled frown. 'Oh, Veronica!' he said, and continued to read, laughing occasionally.

> You refer to my being rude and aggressive to a sister. Was this, I wonder, the occasion when I flung £8000 worth of Hewlett Packard monitoring equipment in the general direction of one of the unit sisters? Well, I must admit that, at first sight this does not give the impression of a friendly gesture, but if you consider my true motives I am sure you will understand. I was actually trying to undermine my colleagues' confidence and create an unpleasant atmosphere within the nursery . . . I am sorry to hear that the sister concerned was admitted to hospital with concussion, but I can assure you it was not the intended result of my action. I must admit that the mood swings to which you refer can be a problem and is not helped by my running around the nursery claiming to be the first Mrs Rochester.

So it went on. Tim finally finished reading and handed it back to me. 'Now that you've vented your fury, go and write something sensible.'

I was lying on the bed when a sudden rap on the door made me jump. I opened it and there was Nick, the first time I had seen him since his return. We went to the interview room where Nick apologised for the can of coke in his hand and asked if I would mind his drinking from it during the interview, as he had been dashing around all day and had not been able to stop for a drink. As seemed usual when I was in Phoenix, the weather was hot and sunny.

He asked me about 'the barney' I'd had at work, saying that Tim had told him something about it. I explained as best I could. Nick asked me what I wanted 'to do about work'. I said that I felt the situation on SCBU was now impossible for me. I had done the best I could and felt I could achieve nothing more there. He agreed, saying that I had 'given Wycombe a bloody good try'. I got the impression that I had given the hoped for answer and he was glad not to need to persuade.

He asked me when I thought I ought to leave them, the ward team. I put my hands in the air in a gesture of consternation. 'Well, I think you got it just about right last time,' Nick responded. I discussed it with Rob later and we decided that I would know when the right time came.

Nick came to see me later, commenting that he had got my letter, and gave a slight laugh. I had sent him a note along with Moira's letter and two replies – one basically representing what I thought of Moira's letter, very frank and uncompromising, and the other, the satirical reply that I had shown Tim.

I remarked that what Moira was saying of me was very strong – she was not just criticising, she was really going in for the attack. Nick agreed with that.

Initially I had wanted to leave as soon as I was permitted, but considering it further I decided that I would wait until Sunday evening. One consideration was the fact that the nursing staff had more time to sit and listen (at least they did then) at a weekend. When Rob approached me and I told him that I had decided to stay until Sunday, he was pleased to hear that I would not be leaving straight away. He said that it would allow them, and me, to prepare properly for my discharge. When I was at home, I missed the nursing input that I received when in hospital.

On Sunday, 6 May 1990, I left hospital after giving the staff a tin of Marks and Spencer biscuits and a card to thank them for their support. I was surprised at how few patients left anything for the staff – on SCBU, we were always being given expensive boxes of chocolates or biscuits, money for the staff fund and even cases of wine. I am sure the work of the staff at Phoenix should be just as much valued as that of a SCBU nurse.

After some time I stopped seeing Vivienne. No one told me why, but there was a suggestion, some years later, that I see her again, though nothing came of that. I later found that she thought my standards were too high and that I was not willing or able to change that. I was apparently too rigid in my thinking. In a letter to a GP, with whom I had just enrolled and whom Nick Rose knew personally, Nick wrote that I 'did not do too well with the uncertainty and lack of structure of psychodynamic work'. He felt that I was sufficiently introspective as it was and that therapies that encouraged introspection were probably not the best thing for me. That was no doubt true, but I did not respond negatively to all types of therapy. I think I responded well to Gilly King in her drama therapy and art therapy sessions – once she had made the effort necessary to induce me to take part in the first instance. In the same letter, Nick wrote that I was quiet and conscientious but that I had a 'recurrent and particularly vicious partially treatment-resistant depression'.

Although it was true that I worked to a very high standard on SCBU, I would argue that it was necessary on a neonatal unit with highly vulnerable babies whose condition could change extremely quickly. In fact, I was not the only nurse there with very high standards. However, I always got on with students, which I do not think would have been so if I had unbendingly high and impossible standards. If things were quiet on the unit, it was to me that the students came asking for teaching. They also liked working with me because, although I expected a reasonable level of performance, I was always aware of their need for encouragement and support.

When I was a third-year student, I was asked to take a student nurse for the day. Each student was being matched up with a staff nurse or third-year student. They were in their initial period of training and this was the first time that they had gone on the ward. At one point in the morning, a tutor from the School of Nursing came and had a chat with my student. When she came back, the student told me that the tutor had said that she was lucky to be with me. Some days later she approached me in the staff dining room and told me that she was the only one not left alone with a patient. I thought that was appalling, as apparently, did the tutors. You might as well have asked someone in from the street to watch your patient. I have no doubt that the patients with whom the students were left were not acutely ill and were not in danger of having a heart attack, but the student would not know that and would probably be left in a state of great anxiety.

From what was put in my notes, you might have thought that I was superior and judgemental, and presumably unpopular as a result. That was not true. I got on well with my colleagues, who liked my sense of humour and were always grateful for my help. This was why Moira's criticism of me as someone who deliberately put people down in their use of technical equipment distressed me so much. When I was first on night duty as the nurse in charge, my night duty colleagues wanted me to ask Moira to put me on nights more often because they liked me being in charge.

It was written in my notes that I thought enrolled nurses were too lowly qualified to work on SCBU. I don't know where that came from, as I have certainly never said it or thought it. We had some very good and competent specialist-qualified enrolled nurses, and I would never have denied that.

I daresay part of the problem of mistakes in my notes was my very quiet speech, which caused people to misunderstand what I was saying. One thing that actually amused me was the utter confusion over who was a sibling or other relative, what their names were and where they lived. Given the number of my friends and relatives and the varying places they lived I suppose this was inevitable – someone wrote that I had a sister called Joan in Crawley – in fact, I had a sister called Jane in Purley. Having said that, I felt it somewhat frustrating after a while. Why could they not get their facts right? I apparently had a sister in Newcastle, then one in Durham – in fact, I had a brother in Carlisle. I could not understand why no one took the simple expedient of drawing a family tree, until Nick did so at the end of 1998.

Chapter 16

I write in reply to Moira's criticism – She is unable to answer
any of my points – Nicholas and Katherine move to Nailsea
– I see occupational health staff, who are sympathetic –
Thoughts – Quote from journal – Discharged but return
to attend groups – Start of problems with Sylvia – Article
published in *Nursing Times*

I began to work on an answer to Moira's diatribe, but it was not
easy. Eventually I came up with the first draft, which I gave to Tim
to read. At one point he drew in his breath. I looked at him quizzic-
ally, so he read, '"You may well have discussed this issue, but if so
it was not with me."' Moira had referred to our having discussed
my 'ability to cope with the type of work on SCBU'. I certainly did
not recall her having referred to that in our conversation, hence the
comment.

So I continued, answering each of her complaints individually
and comprehensively. It took over the space of several weeks to get
to a final draft. Clare persuaded me to be a little more conciliatory
than I was inclined to be, so I changed the last paragraph. I think

she was right in that. I was so furious about the whole thing that the first draft was rather inflammatory.

The reply that I eventually sent said:

17 September 1990

Further to your communication regarding the interview of 9.8.90, you will recall that our discussion centred around events occurring in July, during your recent absence on sick leave. Before considering those points I would like to emphasise my recognition of the support I have received from my colleagues.

Discussion of other matters should not be taken to detract from this.

You refer to particular complaints, but it is difficult for me to respond without further relevant information. I would be grateful for written copies of these complaints, which were presumably taken at the time.

I am surprised at your reference to 'rudeness and aggression', since they are in no way part of my normal behaviour, neither have they been evident as part of my illness. If such a response has been observed on SCBU, I am left wondering why I should behave in such an uncharacteristic manner.

You refer to 'intolerance of many of my colleagues about their capabilities with machinery'. Many colleagues, as I am sure you will agree, have been in the habit of approaching me for technical advice. You yourself did so recently, concerning the Draegar pO_2 monitor; you will recall that my manner was not such as to cause offence.

Indeed, although I have never put myself forward as a technical expert or adviser, I have always responded willingly to requests for help. The fact that people have continued to enlist my advice in these matters suggests that this is true. If I had been anything other than positive and helpful in regard to the use of technical equipment, it would have been most unusual.

I am not, of course, beyond criticism, but I find it difficult to accept some of your comments in their entirety. I cannot agree, for example, that I have a uniform 'general attitude with all staff'. You imply that I have a detrimental effect on 'the morale and feelings of all the parents and whole team of nursing and medical staff'. It is doubtful whether my presence on the unit could have such a profound effect. As you point out, my return to work has been gradual, and I have worked mainly in the cool nursery. During the last eighteen months I have spent unavoidably long absences on sick leave, and once on the unit have had no management role. All these factors limit my influence appreciably. I do not think, given these points, that I can have been the source of the unpleasant atmosphere and lowered morale. This is not lack of insight, simply a judgement of likelihood based on the facts.

You refer to our previously having discussed my 'ability to cope with the work done on SCBU'. You may well have discussed this issue, but I am sure it was not with me. My ability to carry out SCBU work to the required standard has not been in question. You acknowledge in your statement you have given me, that my 'nursing standards are high'.

Finally, you refer to the 'serious nature' of the criticisms. I would certainly agree, and am naturally concerned. It is precisely because of this that I feel I should have been given prior notification of the complaints, and of your intention to discuss them with me. I do not think that it would be considered unreasonable for any member of staff to expect this. I had just returned from two weeks' annual leave and you, owing to your recent sick leave, had not personally seen me at work for about six weeks. I do not feel that it was the ideal time to discuss such issues, especially without warning. I hope you will give consideration, therefore, to the points I have now been able to put forward.

I accept that there may have been times recently when I have not been at my best. If this has caused difficulties to any of my colleagues I deeply regret it. I am sorry if my manner or behaviour has given offence to anyone.

The matter I referred to concerning Moira asking about the Draegar monitor had occurred not long after I had returned to work. Moira had called me into the office where she sat with Ray, head of the electrical engineers department, and his deputy. Ray pointed to two buttons on the Draegar and asked me if there were any other way of switching off the alarm. 'Yes,' I replied, 'the dial at the back.' They each looked at the other and then at me. I began to wonder if I had got it right. After all, it was a while since I had used such technical equipment. I looked at the back of the monitor and was relieved to see the dial I referred to, and pointed it out. Ray looked at it and admitted that he never knew it was there.

I received a somewhat short reply from Moira in which all she did was basically pull rank. The extent of her letter was that it was her duty as senior nurse etc. In fact, she was out of order in what she had said and in the circumstances in which she had said it, as I pointed out in my letter. She did not answer one of the points I had put in my letter, from which I decided that it was safe to assume that she had no answers.

When I was discharged from hospital, I agreed to come back to the ward on Tuesdays and Wednesdays, when I could attend the small group and the women's group. It was decided that I should stay on sick leave from work until I got the situation sorted out, such that I did not have to return to SCBU.

It was soon after that Katherine told me that Nicholas had to change his job location and they were having to move to Nailsea, near Bristol. I was upset to learn this, but realised that they themselves did not want to move. Katherine especially found it hard. I wondered what I would do without them being around.

As regards my job, I went to see Alison Corrigan, one of the tutors at the School of Nursing. I showed her the letter from Moira and explained the problems that I was having on SCBU. I said that I would like to do the Registered Sick Children's Nurse (RSCN) course. She said that there would be no difficulties about a reference from the school. She assured me that they were careful about confidentiality. (I had told her about my experience with personnel.) She then advised me to see occupational health (OH).

At OH I saw Maria, the senior nurse. She was helpful and sympathetic. I was with her for over an hour and we discussed various options. She suggested that I could apply for a vacancy at Wycombe, or elsewhere, through the usual channels. The problem was that I might be rejected on medical grounds if I did not establish my ability to work before applying. Otherwise, I could seek a transfer to another department within Wycombe. Maria said that it would be a shame to waste my specialist skills, though this would limit me to children's or intensive care. There would have to be a vacancy for which I was accepted. Although I would not be going through a normal selection process, I would have to convince another department of my competence.

I gave Maria my version of the dispute with Moira. She commented, 'She obviously sees you as a threat and is not coping with it very well.'

I told her about Moira trying to contact Nick Rose without my consent. She answered that it was very irregular and that no employer should seek to contact an employee's doctor directly. Maria then assured me that I would be consulted and kept fully informed about any approaches they made concerning me and that I was entitled to see written reports about me. Such reports would not be sought without my consent.

Nick's view would be fundamentally important in employers accepting my competence, so Maria suggested that I discuss it with him.

I came out feeling that at last I had found someone in Wycombe who would help me out and did not make me feel that the whole system was against me.

The next time I was due to see Nick, he was off sick so I did not see him until 9 November. I had telephoned Maria to explain the delay. By the time I saw Nick, I had received a letter from Dr Sanderson at OH saying that Moira Campbell had contacted her, asking her to see me. A form for my signature gave OH permission to contact Nick for a report. I was due to see Maria the following Wednesday.

Nick once more instructed me to reduce my dose of amitriptyline by 25 mg, explaining that he wanted to reduce it to a maintenance dose of 100 mg per day.

When I saw Maria again I showed her the letter from Dr Sanderson. She explained that Moira had asked them to see her but given insufficient reason. Dr Sanderson had therefore telephoned SCBU for more information. She told me she would tell me what had been said.

Regarding the form, Maria told me that I would be justified in withholding my signature until I was satisfied of Moira's motives. However, I said that I had no objections to seeing Dr Sanderson, so it seemed reasonable for her to have a report from Nick Rose. I therefore signed the form and left it with Maria.

At about that time I went to a small group meeting in which only Rob, Anne (the occupational therapist), Matt (a psychologist) and one other patient were present. Matt suggested that since few of us were there, it would be a good time to discuss my behaviour in the group. I hardly ever spoke, and when I did I was so quiet that I could hardly be heard. The others all agreed with him and began to criticise. By the end, I was very distressed. Anne came up, put her hand on my shoulder and said she was sorry if what she had said had hurt me. Rob had said the discussion was a waste of time, and she had agreed with him. Matt had disagreed and said that he did not think my behaviour was deliberate. When Rob asked the other patient what he thought, he spoke of his concern about my distress and expressed his sympathy, for which I was grateful.

After the group I stayed in the blue room, very upset. Matt got a coffee and came and sat with me while he drank it. He stayed no more than a few minutes, then left, after expressing his feeling that I did have a real desire to change. He had done that before, bringing his coffee back to the blue room where I was. He usually said nothing other than 'goodbye' before he left but his presence for that time was always a comfort.

Once I had got myself together and entered the quad, the other patient who had been present came to me and asked if I was all right.

Rob went on to night duty and his place was taken by Sylvia. On one occasion in the group I quoted Clare. Clare had recently remarked, 'You're very forgiving.'

Sylvia quickly responded by saying, 'She doesn't know you very well, does she!' I felt irritated that she should question what my own sister, only eighteen months younger than me, had to say of me. I went silent, withdrawing from the discussion. Later Sylvia told one of the other patients that she could not see her as I was in the way. She said nothing to me. I shoved my chair back, pushing myself physically out of the group. I felt that I had been dismissed, though I felt uneasy with myself for cooperating. Later it occurred to me that one could have said that Sylvia caused her own problem, as her chair had been slightly back from the group. Her chair was the misplaced one, not mine. Added to that, why had she not addressed me directly?

In the next small group I had another confrontation with Sylvia when I tried to defend my quote from Clare. I went to that small group feeling better than I had for a while. Matt remarked on it and asked if I could describe the difference in the way I felt. I said that I could think more clearly, did not feel so confused.

There was one organisation in the hospital that I found had a wholly positive effect on me, and that was the Coasters. Oxford remains the only Mental Health Trust to have such an organisation, despite a recommendation from the Commission for Health Improvement, in 2003, that it be replicated nationally. The name Coasters came from the coast-to-coast walk, from St Bees in Cumbria to Robin Hood's Bay in Yorkshire, which was completed every year by a number of service users led by Colin Godfrey, the activities development nurse. Colin runs Coasters, with democratic input from members. No one is ever discharged from Coasters and some members haven't been ill for years, with their involvement in Coasters no doubt aiding their continued good health. Mental health professionals and organisations recognise that physical activity helps to improve mental illnesses such as depression.

I first came into contact with Coasters when I was in hospital and it was suggested to me that some activity would help me, as well as providing a distraction. I began to join the Coasters for badminton on a Tuesday evening, being picked up from the ward and returned later. I continued after being discharged. Coasters also has a regular football team.

The Coasters did not confine itself to Oxford, as Colin had made contact with other Mental Health Trusts. A multi-seated van was bought and painted in the Coasters colours of purple and white, which soon proved its worth. Sports competitions were organised with other Trusts. Colin had been given a substantive post and flexible working hours. Other sports competitors often have to rely on staff giving up free time to lead their teams.

Coasters is not confined to the United Kingdom, as contacts have been made with groups throughout Europe. It was instrumental in forming the European Association of Sport and Social Integration, along with other countries such as Italy and the Czech Republic. This resulted in groups of Coasters travelling in Europe to join in international games. I was able to travel to Italy, a country I had never been to, to join in organised sports. (Well, I took part in the skittles competition.) On the way back we took a two o'clock flight from Pisa, which allowed us time to visit the famous leaning tower. At the time I was not working and was dependent on a benefit. I couldn't have gone to Italy were it not for the Coasters Fund, which paid for my flights and accommodation, all but the £30 I was asked to contribute.

One of the main fund-raising activities for the Coasters is the annual abseil down the John Radcliffe Hospital (JR) in Oxford, which Colin is qualified to supervise. The abseilers are Coasters, carers and members of staff. They do not, I have to confess, include me. You would not get me on the top of the JR, let alone abseiling down it! Others take part in sponsored activities to add to the fund. It does include a contribution from the Mental Health Trust, but that is by no means enough to cover all Coasters activities and other contributions are always welcome. MIND (the mental health charity) has identified a lack of finances as one thing that stands between mental illness sufferers and their ability to engage in physical activity. The Coasters Fund is essential in allowing all members to benefit from organised sport.

Colin remains the only activities development nurse in the country, which is a shame because the Coasters have been highly successful and patients in other Mental Health Trusts would certainly benefit from a similar organisation. The success of Coasters is in no small part owing to Colin himself. He does have a habit of bursting into song when you're in the middle of the Yorkshire moors, with no means of escape, but nobody is perfect. My activities with Coasters have been highly beneficial.

I saw Tim Woodward with the last version of my article. I had mentioned it to Nick Rose. He said that he would be interested to read anything I had written so I left a copy for him with Joy. I thought that he would give it back in passing, with some general comment. In fact, he returned it in the post with a letter. I read the start [his underlining]:

> Many thanks for allowing me to see your article. I think it is extremely powerful, and you should certainly try and get it published.

It continued in an equally complimentary way, and made a few suggestions about what might have been included.

I was surprised, but reminded of my conversation with Tim when I had told him that I was sending it off. I said that it had lost its impact for me and Tim said that it had for him as well but it was still a 'powerful' piece of writing. The time I had given the first version to Tim to read he had come to my room after reading it, literally lost for words. He said, 'I . . . I . . . I almost feel guilty having asked you to write this.' It made me wonder what the *Nursing Times* would make of it.

I next saw Nick Rose on 14 December. He wanted to decrease my dose of amitriptyline to 100 mg, in two stages. He suggested that I reduce it by 25 mg after New Year, since there was a lot to cope with over the festive season.

During Christmas and New Year of 1990–91, I felt generally well. I reduced my amitriptyline dose as Nick had suggested. On 2 January I telephoned Richard, as it was his birthday, but he was not in.

Over the next few days my mood went down and I had some very negative thoughts, which I wrote about in my journal:

> Thoughts and feelings: work – sense of futility. Moira has never valued me – has always tried to put me down, has always opposed me, never encouraged me. I should have realised much earlier and done something about it. Career

non-existent – I'm supposed to be the clever one, I would have been expected to do better than most, not considerably worse. Looking through the *Nursing Times* accentuates those feelings. No point in looking at the jobs – I have no faith in my ability to do them. Paed ITU at the JR advertising – no point in my applying. I couldn't do the job, they would not want me. Feeling generally angry and discouraged. Life is too much like hard work – I wish I could drop dead. If I were to become very depressed again, things would be even more of a mess – the repercussions would be such as to make life unliveable, then there would be no point in attempting to pick myself up off the floor again. Richard – won't commit himself about whether he wants me or not. Hedging his bets, as ever. I wish he'd stop messing me about – I'll have to tell him that.

These thoughts, as ever, drove every normal, positive thought from my mind. Despite this, when I saw Dr Sanderson at occupational health she said that I seemed stronger than when she had last seen me. She said she would write suggesting that I move from SCBU but felt it best not to make any recommendation about where else I might go. I would then have to wait to hear from the hospital. No arrangements were made to see her again but she said that she would be happy to see me if it would help.

Before I left, I went to SCBU. Moira's car was outside but I went in anyway – why should I avoid the place just because of Moira? When I went in, Moira was in the cold nursery. I walked towards the office, waving at Steph in the hot nursery. In the office I spoke to one of my colleagues while I looked to see if there was any post for me. As I walked out I looked studiously ahead, very obviously avoiding meeting Moira's eyes. I surprised myself at the strength of my feelings. Seeing Moira, I felt unable to greet her or to talk to her. If I had realised how strongly I felt, I would not have gone there.

In that week's women's group, I talked about my suicidal thoughts. My failure to take action arose from my not wanting to be dead, Nick had suggested to me, although Tim Woodward disagreed with him on this point. Irreconcilable with Nick's observation but equally valid was my sense of its being right that I should be dead, that I ought to be dead, and that I should therefore kill myself. At home I had been fighting against suicidal feelings that threatened to overwhelm me, so the security represented by hospital, and close observation in Phoenix, gave me a relief that I badly needed. From then on my failure to commit suicide came not from a lack of courage, but from a situation that would not allow it, until I was once again well enough to take responsibility for my own safety.

In saying this, I became very distressed and quite unable to speak. Talking about your feelings of killing yourself is very emotive. I sat rocking myself in my chair. Sylvia commented on this and asked other people in the group if any of them was prepared to respond. One of the patients came over to me, held my hand, then moved closer and put her arm around me. Once she had done this, I broke into tears and began to sob uncontrollably.

Sylvia asked if it felt good to be given permission to cry, and I nodded. Another of the patients came over and put her hand on my arm, speaking sympathetically. When the group ended and we went through to the quad, that patient sat next to me and turned occasionally to put her hand on my arm and say something sympathetic.

I decided to reduce my amitriptyline to 100 mg, disregarding the fact that I had not felt so good lately. I suspected that the causes were independent of my drugs.

Three days later, on a Thursday morning, I visited SCBU, having checked that Moira would not be on duty. She was due on a late shift. I went in and said hello to those in the nursery, then joined Val for a coffee in the sitting room. At about noon I decided to go in case Moira came in early, though it would be unusual for her to come in a full hour and a half early. I went to my locker and took a few things out. I was leaving when I saw Moira at the door of the unit, talking to the senior nurse from the children's ward.

'Oh hello, Veronica, are you going?' she asked.

'Hello. Yes, I'm afraid I am,' I replied.

'Oh!' she said, sounding surprised. 'I want a word. Haven't you got a couple of minutes?'

'No, I'm afraid I haven't. Goodbye.' I responded resolutely.

Moira stood with a look of dismay, and watched me go. I had no intention of subjecting myself to another of Moira's little chats. I did not trust her.

The next day I saw Nick Rose. I told him what had happened on SCBU the previous day. I felt unable to talk with Moira. I also thought, in retrospect, that it would be unwise to talk to her without someone else being present. I asked Nick if I was being reasonable in refusing to talk to Moira. He told me that essentially he thought I was being reasonable in my refusal to speak to her. He commented that encounters with Moira tended to be unpredictable, and that there was really no reason for me to talk to her anyway.

We discussed my medication, Nick commenting that I must be down to 125 mg by now. He was a little surprised when I told him that I had reduced the dose to 100 mg, then said that there was no reason why 100 mg a day should be insufficient. I did explain that I had thought of this in the light of a rather difficult period, but decided that it would not make a difference. He agreed with this.

Not long afterwards I received a letter from the *Nursing Times*, signed by the editor. It said that she would like to accept my article but did not intend to use it for 'quite a while' since they had published several articles on that subject recently. I had wondered whether they would refuse my article because of this. However, the magazine said that they would publish the article if I accepted that they would not do so immediately. I wrote back agreeing to this and enclosing two new paragraphs that I suggested should replace the first paragraph of the original piece. This change came about through my considering a point made by Nick Rose – that the natural point of entry to my subject was the problems a health worker has in accepting that they have an emotional problem requiring specialist help. I decided that I agreed with this, and that it contributed more to the discussion than the original opening.

On Tuesday, 26 February 1991, I saw Mrs Newman, patient services manager at High Wycombe Hospital. Also present were Linda from personnel (who had inspired me with distrust the previous August when Moira had arranged for me to see her), and Mr Davies from the Royal College of Nursing.

Mrs Newman quoted from a letter she had received from Dr Sanderson saying that, in the interests of my health, I should not return to SCBU. She asked if there was anything I would like to say about what she had read. I said first, that it had never been suggested that work on SCBU was not appropriate for me, that leaving SCBU was not because I was not suited to the work, and that I intended to return to that type of work. Secondly, regarding other matters, I said I did not wish to discuss them at that point; I did not wish to get involved with them in the interests of my health.

Mrs Newman accepted this, though I wondered if she were fishing for something in her question. We discussed the question of where I would go on my return. I suggested the children's ward but Mrs Newman was dubious about this because of changes taking place there. I said that I was prepared to return to adult nursing, although I had been on SCBU ever since I had qualified. I had nursed adults before and I could do it again.

The matter of how to reorientate me into working again and how my progress should be monitored, was raised. I commented that I would be quite happy to accept some form of monitoring, adding that an unfortunate aspect of what had happened the previous August was the sudden nature of the criticisms put to me. I expressed the view that the whole episode had been entirely unnecessary. I added that I assumed Mrs Newman had read the relevant correspondence. She said that she had not, since my personnel file had been lost. It was only when I was going home that it occurred to me that I had been told my personnel file was missing when I saw Linda on Thursday, 9 August 1990; the first communication from Moira purported to be the record of an interview on 7 August, and was dated 9 August. The absence of copies of the correspondence between Moira and myself could not be explained by the loss of a file that occurred before 9 August. It also occurred to me that two letters praising my actions in handling a situation on SCBU, from Mrs Newman herself and Mr Collier, acting unit general manager, would have been in the file that had so unfortunately been lost. Helen Carter, the maternity manager, had telephoned me at the time to ask if she could save a copy of my statement as an example of how to write one. No doubt it would have been inconvenient to have those on my record, given the circumstances.

I received a letter dated 5 March, which went over the basis for our discussion. Mrs Newman said that she found my 'realistic approach to the discussion both helpful and constructive'. She went on to decide that children's ward was the best place for me to go, and suggested that I return three days a week initially, using up my annual leave. She awaited confirmation from me that this was acceptable, and that I was considered fit to return to work.

I next saw Nick ten days later. The letter from Mrs Newman gave a fairly comprehensive description of what had happened, and how the situation was, so I gave it to him to read. He commented that the tone of the letter was encouraging and I agreed. He asked if I thought I was ready to return to work. I replied that I thought it was time I got back, though the prospect was rather daunting. The only thing was to get back there and get into it.

We ran out of time before I could raise the matter of the groups, and I wondered if that was just as well. I was tentative about complaining to a doctor about a nurse.

Sylvia had taken over from Rob, who was on night duty, so she was in the small group as well as the women's group. Her theory was that I had an antipathy towards female authority figures and that this explained all my difficulties. She also stated that I saw her as a female authority figure. This was a very neat theory – my very disagreement with her, interpreted as antagonism towards her, seemed to prove the theory.

I did not accept that I regarded Sylvia as a female authority figure – she represented authority no more than any of the other female nurses in Phoenix, with whom I had no problems. Indeed, you could say that Sylvia represented authority no more than I did when at work. I was the last person to see a staff nurse as an authority figure.

Sylvia based her theory on my reaction to two people – Moira and herself. I did point out to Sylvia that she did not know anything about my response to other female authority figures – she did not even know how many I had come across in the course of my life. At another time I pointed out that I had spent seven years in a convent school with no problems, but Sylvia replied that a convent was probably the best place to learn to resent female authority figures, and added that she knew because she had been to one. I felt that she was being flippant, but I could not respond. I did think that if Sylvia had been to a convent and that if that was the best place to learn the resentment of female authority figures, then she was practically admitting to having such problems herself. Perhaps she was putting her problems on to me? After all, I had said, quite truthfully, that I had never had any difficulties at the convent so it cannot have had that affect on me – I would surely have had problems with the nuns if I had resented them.

I was feeling increasingly threatened and frustrated by the situation. I was aware of failing to put across my viewpoint comprehensively or effectively. Sylvia repeatedly complained that she could not hear me because I faced downwards (which was true) and spoke quietly. One of the reasons for this behaviour was, I think, that I felt threatened and was withdrawing into myself, putting up the barriers to protect myself. I felt that I was constantly under attack from Sylvia and I was beginning to wonder if she was doing this deliberately. I felt uncertain about trusting her – I was always wondering what she was up to.

Sylvia kept drawing attention to the effort I put into controlling my emotions. In this she was quite right, and I was left wondering how important this was. I did not feel safe enough in the groups to ever contemplate losing that control. I felt attacked and besieged. I often, too often, became distressed in the groups, but always put all I could into keeping the situation under control. As Sylvia once commented, I even cried in a controlled manner. (I was, it was true, a person of extreme self-control. I remember driving with my brother-in-law in the car. 'Cor! What self-control!' he said. 'Keeping to thirty when there is a clear straight road ahead of you.')

One Tuesday I saw Mrs Newman and accordingly missed the small group. I deliberately telephoned Phoenix so that there would be the best chance of ensuring that Sylvia (who would be on that afternoon) would get the message. I telephoned in the morning of the meeting and at handover time when most nursing staff would be in the office. I was familiar with Phoenix communications, which usually went awry. As it was, the message did not get to Sylvia – at least, she said nothing about having received it.

I missed the next group because I was a couple of minutes late. Groups often started up to ten minutes late. The group could hardly have started but I did not want to walk in on my own and interrupt. I went for a walk then sat in my car for a while before returning to Phoenix.

In the next women's group I attended, Sylvia asked me why I had not been at the last week's women's group. I do not remember what I replied – my memory of what happened in the groups was becoming frustratingly unreliable. Sylvia referred to my sitting out in my car as being 'provocative' (maybe she was right). She had once described my speaking quietly as 'arrogant'. (She was wrong there – my voice went quieter the more threatened or vulnerable I felt.)

When she asked why I was absent from the women's group, I felt accused. I said that I had good reason to miss the women's group, and might have added that it was nothing to do with missing the small group the next day. Sylvia, inevitably but inaccurately, connected the two absences. I made no further explanation. Why bother? It would not make any difference.

In the small group Matt commented, 'We missed you last week.'

That night I decided that I could not face the groups any more. I went into Phoenix and told Tim, but after our conversation I agreed to give the groups one more try. I was not happy giving up, as if I were running away, just because someone was saying something that I did not want to hear. Tim suggested that I tell Sylvia of my decision. I saw her in the office. She commented that I seemed not to be feeling so good. I was surprised at this comment. She said that she would be on annual leave for two weeks and would see me afterwards. When she returned to the groups I quoted Sylvia as saying that I had returned to the groups because I did not want to be beaten by her. She denied having said that but commented that it was important I had thought she had said it.

Things did not improve, however, and eventually I decided, reluctantly, that the only solution was to withdraw from the groups. Apart from anything else, the attitude of the other nurses was that I should solve the problem with Sylvia. They were obviously not prepared to give me any support.

Despite the sympathetic support of Matt, who once told Sylvia in a group that she had gone too far with me, I could cope no longer. It cost me much to admit this, but I felt that I could not manage Sylvia's apparent hostility any more. I wrote a note to Sylvia, thinking carefully about what to write, as I wanted to write words that she could not make something of. I cannot remember exactly what I wrote, except that I said I felt 'profoundly unsafe' in the groups. For me it was a failure, and I felt it keenly, but I felt that I had no alternative.

Meanwhile, I considered my return to work. I did wonder about the senior nurse of children's ward. I remembered the time I saw her chatting with Moira outside SCBU. She must have heard Moira's version of the necessity for my move. In practice, however, you would have thought that she had known nothing of me in advance. I got on very well with all the staff on the ward, especially Nicola, who was given the task of being my mentor. I actually enjoyed my time on Ward Seven.

It was while I was on the ward that my article was finally published in the *Nursing Times* of 4–10 September 1991, under the title 'Real nurses don't go mad', which was, I decided once I'd thought about it, quite a good title. Mrs Newman knew about it before its publication. In fact, she had come to me and said, 'Are you sure you want to put your name to this? I've been careful to keep secret what's been wrong with you.' Secret, I noted, not confidential. I suspected that if I, as a High Wycombe nurse, had had an article published on another subject she would have been all too pleased. It reminded me of Moira and her comment, 'after all, you have suffered a *mental* illness'. One did not confess to having had a mental illness.

To my surprise, a letter came all the way from Denmark. It was written by a Danish nurse tutor who told me that she was so affected by it that she had translated it for her students. Another came from a Samaritan counsellor, who asked me if I had any more of my writing that I could let him have. He, likewise, expressed how he had been very affected by it. I remembered the comment that Nick had made about its being 'extremely powerful'.

Tim telephoned me at the ward to congratulate me.

On the day of my article's publication I was in the office with several other members of the staff having a coffee break when Pat, the ward clerk, came in the door, looked at me and raised a copy of the *Nursing Times*. She came over and said to me, 'I never knew you had had such a terrible experience.' She then went on to ask me what I would like them to do – would it help if they talked about it, or did I prefer that they not say anything about it? I had to admit I was not sure, but I was really grateful for her sympathetic and sensitive response. I had been very open and descriptive about what I had been through and I have to admit that I was in a state of trepidation about something so very personal being made public. I was, however, discovering the widespread attitude that mental illness was something you should keep secret, to use Mrs Newman's word. I had come to believe strongly that those with mental illness suffered all the more for being regarded as part of such an occult subject.

I had not received a copy of the objectives that Mrs Newman had for me, but Nicola and the senior nurse both had copies 'so they know what you're doing'. I telephoned Mrs Newman's office to be told that they had had no instructions to give me a copy. Given my recent experiences, this made me somewhat suspicious. When I saw her, Mrs Newman assured me that she had intended me to have a copy. I facetiously commented that I wondered if it was by way of making it official that I did not know what I was doing. This comment was taken seriously and I was assured that that was not what she meant. Perhaps I should have asked her precisely what she did mean.

Chapter 17

One way out of this situation, I decided, was to work towards something that I had long thought of achieving, and to apply for my Registered Sick Children's Nursing course. I started investigating the possibilities. Dr Sanderson and my GP were very encouraging. I had not yet spoken to Nick but Nicola considered it a good idea She suggested that I should tell Mrs Newman, who would probably be pleased.

Mrs Newman was not pleased – in fact, she advised me against applying at that time. She was rather vague, so I asked her specifically what her reasons were. Even then she did not give me a straight answer. She mentioned Moira Campbell and her saying that I had been moved from the department.

I was pretty dumbfounded by this response so left without further comment.

If anything Mrs Newman had heard or seen had led her to regard my move from SCBU as anything other than medical, why had I not been told? After all, she claimed not to have seen the correspondence between Moira and me.

Dr Sanderson was as encouraging and supportive as ever. She agreed that the reasons for the move, officially, were purely medical. She read from Nick Rose's letter in which he was careful not to make the nature of the medical problem clear, so allowing for the letter to be quoted. 'He doesn't actually say it, but we know what he means,' Dr Sanderson commented. She said that Moira should be writing a reference regarding my performance before I was ill, and added that my illness was for Nick, herself and my GP to comment on. I had not spoken to Nick but she recommended that I do so. When I explained the situation to him, he said that he thought I should not hold back 'just because some people chose not to be helpful'.

I contacted the RCN representative, who was helpful and pointed out that there was no reason why I should not ask someone other than Moira to write a reference.

Near the end of the allocation I had to see Mrs Newman and Nicola, with the report she had been asked to write. I think Nicola was more worried about that report than I. Originally, when asked by Mrs Newman to give a report on how I had managed, Nicola had spoken with the senior sister. They agreed that I was doing well and they could see no problems, and told Mrs Newman so. She said that it was not good enough and poor Nicola ended up having to write a lengthy and comprehensive report according to detailed criteria that Mrs Newman provided.

I should not have been surprised when I did not receive a copy of the report. I kept on telephoning Mrs Newman's office, the first excuse from her staff being that she had not told them to give me a copy. I was not going to take that this time. I pointed out that I had a right to see the report. It must have been about that time that I relieved my feelings by writing 'The hospital manager's guide to the rehabilitation of lunatics' –

Literature: careful reading of Machiavelli's *The Hospital Manager* is recommended . . .

Equipment: shredder for shredding records you lost yesterday . . .

By the time of the meeting to discuss the report, my efforts had been in vain so I simply stated to Mrs Newman, as I stood outside her office, that I was not prepared to discuss a report that I had not read. 'But this meeting was arranged to discuss the report,' she replied, indignantly. I repeated myself. She was not amused – but I doubt that she was as angry as I.

In fact, the report was really very good and any adverse comments (about which Nicola was apologetic) I admitted were fair. What sort of honest report on anyone could be wholly good? Anyway, those points that were adverse (and they were only mild and infrequent) suggested that the report was accurate and I could take the good points as truth. Mrs Newman allowed me to comment in writing on the eight-page report 'briefly'.

Just over a month after this I put my plan of escape into action by going to the Hospitals for Sick Children, Great Ormond Street (GOS), for an interview. I was delighted and almost in disbelief when I was told that I had a place. I was inevitably referred to OH. The doctor did not want to see me then but in April, when I had been out of hospital for eighteen months. I was informed that the school would be told of the decision to see me but not the reason. Another scrupulous and unprejudiced OH department. In April 1992, I left High Wycombe hospital for the final time. On Thursday, 27 April 1992, I started my RSCN course in London.

On 12 August I saw my GP (I had not yet transferred to a London GP), who did not think that I was in a fit state to go to work. When I said that I was all right, he said, 'You're *not* all right. You're as bad as I've ever seen you.' I was admitted, in Nick's absence, by his SHO, an authoritative but actually quite sensitive doctor who proved to be very supportive. I prevaricated, however, despite being threatened with a section at one point. I was not actually admitted until 27 August. That admission was of particular significance for me, as when Nick returned, he told me that he had been thinking of replacing lithium with MAOIs (monoamine oxidase inhibitors, they act on brain chemicals, as do other antidepressants) or ECT. He recommended the latter because it would take time to effect the drug changeover, whereas ECT would have an immediate effect. Nick did, however, assure me that he would respect my decision. After several days, I finally conceded. What else could I do? Nick knew that ECT was anathema to me, and I was sure that he would have taken my antipathy into account in deciding to recommend that treatment.

In the circumstances, I decided that I would have to sign a consent form and put myself in the care of the ECT department staff, who proved very good, and sympathetic to my anxieties. I had to walk down to the ECT department, which was in a small building at the bottom of the courtyard in the old hospital. Once we moved across the road to the new hospital, there was a new, modern department in the same building as the ward. The nurse accompanying me carried my medical notes. I asked her if she would stay with me and she assured me that she would.

There was another lady having ECT that morning but she was not at all worried about it, so the nurses decided to take me in first since I was in a state of some anxiety. The staff in the department soon got to know me and always ensured that I went in first. They had advised that I wear loose clothing. I was asked to take off my shoes and climb up onto a trolley and lie down. I remembered that when I had had meningitis, they had wheeled me around the hospital lying flat on a trolley and I had not liked it then. It made me feel helpless, and when I was wheeled into the ECT room I felt supremely so.

Nurses and doctors moved around me, putting monitors on and checking equipment. I felt like sitting up and demanding to know what they were doing, though in reality I knew. An anaesthetist managed to place a cannula first time, which was a relief because doctors often had trouble getting access to my veins. I do not like anaesthetics at the best of times, but being aware that electric shocks will be sent through your brain once you are unconscious made it particularly hard for me to tolerate.

I became aware of what was happening once again when seated in a chair in a sitting room. The nurse who had accompanied me from the ward offered me a cup of tea. I was so confused that I thought I was still nil by mouth, so I refused it. I asked them next time to tell me when I had woken up following the treatment, so that I could get my bearings. That was something else the ECT nurses got used to when dealing with me.

I suffered from short-term memory loss, but I began to recall things a matter of hours afterwards. It certainly had a positive effect on my depression, but I didn't like it any better afterwards than I did before – perhaps even less. On subsequent admissions, when Nick once more felt ECT to be so necessary as to override my antipathy, I would agree to the treatment. I did not like it and Nick knew that I did not, such that I had confidence in his taking that into account in any decision to use ECT.

I never became entirely reconciled to ECT, however. When I was in hospital in 1996, I was in a particularly distressed state. I walked through main reception followed by Julie, one of the nurses. I told her that everyone would be better off without me. She argued against this. I had had my car keys in my hand throughout this and now got into my car, locking the doors. At this point one of the nurse managers came out of the hospital to go home. She stayed where she was, suggesting that Julie go for help. She tried to talk to me, but I would not cooperate so she went to her car, going home, or so I thought. In fact, she drove it in front of mine so that I could not go anywhere. Julie then returned with Rory, another nurse.

The nurse manager persuaded me to wind down my window a little, so that she could better talk to me. It actually allowed her to put her hand in and unlock the door, so that Julie could take the keys out of the ignition. I was annoyed with myself for being stupid enough to allow this. The manager went home.

Eventually I was persuaded to get out of the car, realising that I could go nowhere. I went to reception with Julie, but refused to go to the ward. Rory stayed to lock up the car.

I felt that I had messed things up by not acting on my suicidal feelings when I could have done. There was a message saying that Nick was on the ward and wanted to see me, but I said that he should go home and leave me. A message came back that he would come out and see me. I told Julie to tell him not to. She said that he had been planning to see me anyway, but I felt sure she was just saying that. I spoke to Julie and Rory, and they were both sympathetic. Julie told me to tell Nick all that I had told her. The task of going over it all again seemed immense.

Nick turned up soon after with a demeanour suggesting that nothing untoward was happening, rather than that I was being a nuisance and keeping him back when he should have been on his way home. He took me to a side room and Rory returned to the ward.

Nick started by expressing his surprise that I had apparently taken a turn for the worse and asked if anything specific had happened to cause it. I replied that nothing had happened and could not express what was wrong, or give an explanation. Nick then suggested that he say what he thought was happening. The effect of the ECT I had had, he thought, had worn off. In addition, I had stopped the venlafaxine I was on and could not start the new drug until the Monday, so I had nothing to hold me up. He said that he thought he should have tried harder to persuade me to continue the ECT.

We talked for quite a while. I expressed how I felt about my failure to end things, yet again. He said that he thought, deep down, I did not want to take that course. I replied that that was the problem, otherwise I would have done something effective. Maybe I did not want to, but whenever those feelings came into my mind I had a strong feeling of *ought* to. He said that the decisions I had actually taken were the right ones. I replied that they did not feel right, and caused me great pain. Nick acknowledged that, but said he thought that the decision I did make, to go on struggling with the depression, was the more courageous.

On ECT, Nick was respectful of my feelings. He said there was nothing magical about it, that it was just a way of influencing neurotransmitters, which was, after all, no more manipulative of the brain than were drugs, and if anything the side-effects were fewer. Eventually he gave me his usual reassuring squeeze of the shoulder, then took me back to the ward. He went to the clinical room to write me up a drug to calm my thoughts, then returned to my room. He told me to think about ECT, 'but don't worry about it'.

After he had gone, Julie came with 4 mg trifluorperazine, saying that Dr Rose had sent it and that I could take as much or as little as I liked. I swallowed the lot, as I was distressed and desperate for as complete a relief as possible. Nick later commented on how I really had been in quite a dreadful state.

Nick came to see me on the Wednesday. He said that he thought it was time to increase the antidepressant moclobemide as my mood had dropped. He then asked me to consider having another ECT on Friday, as he felt that I needed it. I reminded him that, back in 1989, I had said that no one had told me that the depression of my teenage years might return. At one point it had looked as if the depression might go away, as it had when I was a teenager, but it had not. Indeed the depression kept on returning and I never knew when it would do so. I said that I did not want to face a future so subject to depressive phases.

Nick replied that I had every right to make that decision but it was his duty to make sure that I did not make it when influenced by depression. I told Nick that I did not see why he did not leave me to my own devices, but he said that he was committed to treating me and would not give up.

I spent several days that week trying to decide whether to consent to ECT on the Friday. When I was asked about it on Wednesday, I expressed my uncertainty. Earlier in the week I had been sure that I would not, but by then I could hardly express any coherent view. I felt completely confused.

On Friday morning, no one came into my room. No one asked me if I wanted my drugs. It seemed to me that they had simply decided to go ahead without worrying what I thought and I began to feel quite angry about that. It was getting towards 10.00 and I expected that the next thing to happen would be the arrival of a nurse to take me to ECT.

At that point someone did arrive, but it was not a nurse. It was Nick Rose, who explained that he had left the ward round to talk to me about whether I would agree to have ECT that morning. I could only shrug my shoulders and shake my head in a confused manner. I did not know what to say, though I was grateful he had come to achieve some resolution. He said he appreciated how difficult it was to make decisions at such times, as I could only continue to express complete uncertainty. He gave me some time, then said, 'Shall we go ahead then?' I nodded.

On another occasion the nurses actually forgot that there was the likelihood of my having ECT that morning and someone brought me a cup of tea. Nick came to talk to me about ECT. He finished by saying that his senior house officer (SHO) would come to see me with a consent form. He left, taking with him the tea and an apple that were by my bed. The nurse came in soon after and apologised for bringing the tea, asking me if I had drunk any. I admitted that I had taken a mouthful, but that was apparently not enough to prevent me from having an anaesthetic.

When the SHO came, he asked me if I understood why Dr Rose had recommended ECT. 'All the classic reasons,' he said, 'suicidal thoughts, the general biology, motor retardation.' It was not only the mood but the physical signs of depression which I displayed that made my case appropriate for ECT. He said little other than that. I signed the form.

I was in hospital twice during my course at GOS, which caused real difficulties. The first admission, when I had ECT, was two months long and the second, one month. The second time, when Nick first came to see me in my room, he remarked, 'I guess you must be very angry with yourself for being here.'

At the beginning of that admission, GOS asked me to sign a resignation form, which I did, because it was easiest to do that and I could not cope with considering it rationally. Nick Rose considered that I was in no fit state of mind to make such a decision, and my lack of consideration no doubt demonstrated that. I was determined to finish my course, despite all, so I took up a post as a charge nurse in a nursing home, as that was the only place where I could find a temporary but sufficiently responsible post. I would complete the course somehow. As it was, I managed to persuade the course tutor to take me back and I earned my precious RSCN.

When I was in Phoenix there were other groups in progress, apart from the small group and the women's group, such as the drama group, which had totally terrified me during my initial admission. I would pace up and down the blue room as far away as I could get from the activity. It was run by an occupational therapist called Gilly, who expended a great deal of patience and understanding in gradually getting me involved. Years afterwards I continued to feel extremely reserved in the drama group but Gilly could always manage to get me to join in. I actually found it to be one of the most helpful of the groups that I attended. Gilly also managed art therapy, which I found helpful as well.

I have never received medical treatment to the exclusion of the so-called 'talking treatments', which has so often been the complaint of psychiatric patients. Vivienne found me an unsuitable candidate for CBT. I also took part in various kinds of group therapy, of course. Each of the counsellors I had I found helpful, though some were easier than others to get used to.

While I was in London I went to Oasis, a counselling service recommended by the OH doctor, who had also suggested that I enrol myself with the local practice of Dr Morrison. My counsellor, Mr B, sometimes caused me difficulties. I have never known someone quite so unsmiling, even on meeting after I had been seeing him for many months, and I found it a bit off-putting. He proved to be quite insightful at times, though I sometimes found what he said difficult to cope with, and it could make me feel frustrated or angry. He usually commented on such responses.

He appeared to be quite interested in my relationship with Sylvia, as well he might. One day he commented that I felt angry when I did not get the response that I was looking for – and he cited Sylvia – saying that I looked for help from group therapy. 'Was that not what it was for?' I said. He replied, very pointedly, 'Exactly'. One day he said that I was using the reasonable side of me to punish what I saw as my unreasonable side – I had called myself absurd and unreasonable. He suggested that I thought I did not deserve attention and found it difficult to accept – in response to my problems I seemed to be 'tearing myself apart'. I understandably found him quite challenging.

I had told him about my leaving the groups. I had also told Nick Rose, deliberately not naming Sylvia, why I had abandoned the groups. However, Nick soon observed, 'We are talking about Sylvia here, aren't we?'

I went on but said little other than the basic facts. He said that perhaps I should think about what Sylvia had been suggesting. This, of course, was not what I wanted to hear. Mr B suggested that I was deliberately avoiding talking about Sylvia with Nick again, because I was afraid that I would be angry with him. I realised that it was now two years since I had left the groups and the spectre of Sylvia continued to haunt me. I could not get away from all those problems I had experienced in her groups.

I decided that I would have to see Nick about it again. The nurses had failed me completely, making clear that it was a problem between Sylvia and I in the groups and that they had no intention of intervening. When I thought about it, I had given Nick little to go on. I had given basic facts but no real idea of the affect she was having on me. I did my usual thing of being as neutral as possible and carefully avoiding emotion. Mr B was right. I was afraid of getting angry with Nick, or perhaps his not believing me so that I fell in his estimation. His faith in me and support of me were important. I did not want to lose them.

I admitted from the start that I was talking about Sylvia and about her insistence that I should think about her theory. I pointed out that she, with her feedbacks, handovers, chats over a cigarette and behind office doors, had had her view considered quite enough, whereas I had been denied a chance to put forward my view. I went on to give him a detailed and completely honest account of what had happened and what I felt about it. I fully expressed my anger and frustration and said that someone ought to have done something. Nick asked if he should have done something. I considered this, then said it had been a problem with the nursing staff and they should have done something. Nick commented that he did not realise at the time what was happening. This did not surprise me – groups tend to be perceived as a nursing provenance.

I was with Nick almost an hour, during which time he listened with total respect for what I was saying. For the first time someone simply listened to what I had to say. By the time I got to the end, I was tearful and distressed. Nick acknowledged that there was some very strong emotion there, adding that the question was what to do about it. He asked me if I wanted to make a formal complaint but I said no. He said that he hoped I would not need to go back into hospital, but if I did then this problem would have to be taken into account. He could certainly feed back my feelings to Sylvia and acknowledged that there was no point in my doing that. He asked me what I wanted him to do. I said I most wanted to know what had happened. I wanted to know why I was refused help and support. I wanted to know what was being said about me to come to the decision to reject and abandon me. One of the things that angered me most was the way I was kept out of all discussions on the decision for me to be rejected and abandoned. I had been given no feedback, so that I was left feeling confused and frustrated. In response to this Nick reminded me that I could get a copy of my notes. When I did so, I found that Sylvia had documented nothing on the matter. It was as if all those troubles had never occurred. She most certainly should have documented them, and not to do so was a dereliction of duty.

As I went through the door I paused and apologised to Nick, saying that I seemed to have spent the whole session moaning at him. He commented that that was all right, we knew each other well enough by then.

I went away feeling as if a load had been taken away. I was

incredibly relieved. He had taken me seriously, listened to me, recognised and acknowledged the genuineness of my feelings and suggested what could be done to help.

The staff in Phoenix continued, in all other matters, to be a great source of support. I had some very good named nurses. I always liked, if possible, to have the same named nurse on subsequent admissions. The person who was my named nurse for the greatest length of time was Tim Ackland, who had a great sense of humour and had an entirely inoffensive way of being almost constantly cheerful. The old hospital having been sold (and turned into rather expensive apartments), a new hospital was built across the road. Before it was opened the nurses were given an opportunity to look around it. Tim came back and said how great it was. Single, carpeted rooms with fitted wardrobes, bedside lights and a wash basin. 'Just like Tescos!' he declared. When I saw the building, I could see what he meant – modern, one-storey building with a little tower at the top.

This did not prevent him from attending to serious matters. I was always one who wanted to know exactly what was happening and being said. Nick was good about that, but I have to say that not all the nurses were. Tim Ackland, however, always asked me before a ward round if there was anything I wanted him to ask. Afterwards

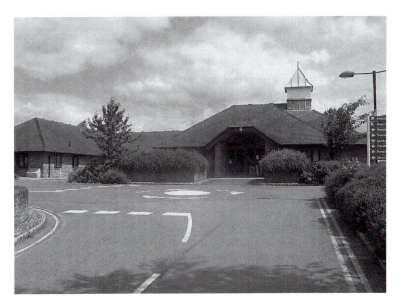

Figure 17.1 The new Littlemore Mental Health Centre, with its little tower at the top – 'just like Tescos'

he would find me to tell me what had happened in the round and what had been said about me. Often I had to search around for hours to get a particular piece of information from other nurses.

Another named nurse, Sandra Young, became ward manager, when she continued her care of me, then left to work in the community where I was lucky enough to have her as a community psychiatric nurse (CPN). I have always found my CPNs very helpful and supportive. The one thing I missed about not being in hospital, a state otherwise entirely to be commended, was the lack of nursing input. This was solved by having a CPN. My present CPN, Tim Cole, has been with me for a while. He has helped me to make the recent transition from one consultant to another. An experienced mental health nurse is a highly competent professional; although I have inevitably come across some with whom I have had a less than therapeutic relationship, the majority have been caring and sensitive.

The SHO who admitted me for my first hospitalisation while at GOS had asked me, 'Why have you never been sectioned? Have you had pressure put on you or have you been too ill?' I admitted that it had been both.

I had seventeen admissions from 1989 until July 2008, ranging in length from a few weeks to six months. Until 2005 I had never been under a section. I spent Christmas 2005 in hospital under section. I can remember practically nothing about what happened because I was given so much ECT. A nurse told me that I had been 'practically catatonic'. Apparently I refused food, drink and any treatment and Nick Rose decided that I did not have the capacity to make my own decisions. He wrote in my notes that I needed ECT 'to save life and for humanitarian reasons'. The latter was in recognition of the pain and distress caused by severe depression. All that I know of that period I have gleaned from what others say, my own journal – in which I seemed to have written something at the time – and my medical records, which I requested.

I do remember one other occasion when Nick was insistent that I be admitted. I asked what would happen if I refused and he told me that there would be a tribunal of three, one of whom would be a doctor who did not know me. He did not know what they would decide. I did not want to be sectioned. 'I haven't got any choice, have I?' I commented.

'No,' he said gently, 'you haven't got any choice.' I accepted admittance to hospital.

Following a seminar at a MIND conference, I decided to write an advance directive stating what I wished to be done if I were mentally unfit to make my own decisions. I recorded in it instructions to ensure that my little dog was cared for (important things first), those persons who were to be informed of my admission – I named next of kin, though legally I did not have that power. I registered my well-known antipathy to ECT. Nick asked if I would write a short article on advance directives for the *Psychiatric Bulletin*, so that other psychiatrists could have the patient's view, so I did. He sent it off and it was published in October 2002.

I have been known to resist admission until Nick has said, 'If you can't make the decision, I will,' then reminded me of the advance directive. In retrospect, in a more reasonable state of mind, I have had to admit that he has been right.

Admitting a patient who is seriously ill, without a section, is felt to be unfair by MIND and other such interested parties, on the grounds that a patient compromised by mental illness does not get the protection of tribunals and such legal securities, unless they are sectioned. I preferred, however, to trust to those who knew me and my illness best, and to avoid sections.

Sylvia had told me that the doctor who had asked me why I had never been sectioned 'was on the verge of sectioning you'. In the context, I did not know how to take it.

I have many times been aware that I have been on the edge of sectioning. I remember one occasion, when I had left the ward, I was parked in a barely used little track when a police car drew up and two officers, concerned at my being there on my own, approached me to see if I was all right. They mentioned that they came from Watlington, which would explain why they did not know me. The ward would have informed the Oxford police. One policeman sat back on his heels beside me, while the other moved away, speaking into his radio. They were both very patient with me, although they often had to ask me to repeat myself as I spoke so quietly. They asked me where I came from.

'Littlemore,' I said with all honesty.

'That's the mental health unit, isn't it?' the second officer remarked, slipping my keys out of the ignition and putting them into his pocket. The first continued to talk to me. He was called away by his colleague to talk to whoever was on the radio. He then returned and sat on his heels beside me again. He said, 'Now I'm going to take you back and I am giving you no choice. I'm going to take you back, okay?'

Those who have never been depressed themselves find it hard to take suicidal thoughts seriously. However, such thoughts are greatly disturbing. I spent a weekend driving around the countryside, stopping in quiet lay-bys at night, with all my drugs – enough to kill me, said my knowledge of drugs – a large bottle of water and a suicide note. These were all pointers to serious intent. I telephoned Nick Rose a few times but refused to tell him where I was. What I needed was to talk to someone who would take what I told them seriously but would stay calm. Each time I telephoned he would tell me when he would be at Littlemore, though he commented that he did not know how far away I was, and therefore how long it would take me to get there. I did not give him this information, yet at no point was I more than five miles from Oxford. When I finally walked into his office, knowing when he had said he would be there, I confessed about the drugs and the bottle of water I had put in the car before I left home and the suicide note I had written. He remarked, 'I think that's a measure of how desperate you have become.'

There are some who simply do not believe your obsessive thoughts, while others believe them but do not know what to do. Sometimes those persons can be yourself.

In the period preceding my going away in my car, I had spoken to Tim Woodward a couple of times. He recognised that I was becoming deeply depressed. In fact, he became sufficiently concerned to write a piece in my notes, so as to ensure that Nick knew of his concerns. Tim (who was a CPN by then) told me later that he had not written in my notes since I was a patient in the old Phoenix.

The standard verdict in the case of suicide is that the person acted 'while the balance of their mind was disturbed'. This is not said simply to make it sound better. A great many suicides are suffering from a psychiatric condition, usually depression, and they are not acting in their right minds. My behaviour was certainly not normal when I was seriously ill, suicidal or not. The patience of the nurses, which I tried greatly at times, was amazing.

On one occasion I arrived on the ward and asked to speak to Julie, who took me to one of the interview rooms. She was very sympathetic when I attempted to explain how I felt. Eventually I broke into tears. Julie said that she would get the doctor to see me. This, as usual, left me feeling confounded. What did I want a doctor for?

The ward SHO had a rather one-sided conversation with me, as I went quiet on him. It was then put to me that I should be in hospital. I said that I was going home. Julie commented that I had realised something was wrong and had done the right thing by coming to them. I was then told that there were no beds free in Phoenix and I would be admitted to Wintle, at the Warneford Hospital. That made me more determined. I demanded my car keys, which Julie had taken. I then declared that, if they did not let me have my keys, I would get the bus. I was then somehow persuaded to go and sit outside reception at Phoenix.

At some point I decided to leave. The doctor and a nurse caught up with me just as I reached the hospital exit. The nurse stood in front of me and moved to obstruct me whenever I tried to go around him. I had no choice but to return to the ward with them. Not long after, I left again – this time by the small sluice and the door they used to put the waste bags out. I went out of the hospital and was walking towards the village when the nurse who had come after me before, along with another nurse, caught up with me. 'Come on, Veronica,' he said, 'we can't go doing this all evening. Here, take my hand.' At first I refused but, having once more realised that I would not be allowed to go any further, I put my hand in his. He led me safely over the road, which I had crossed without bothering to look for traffic, then let go of my hand and walked beside me. 'Let's go back and discuss the options,' he said. When we got back, he left as the night shift came on.

Sylvia was on that night and sat behind the desk in the office. The doctor was there also. I sat outside, getting increasingly angry and agitated. Finally, I flung open the office door, marched in and demanded my keys, stating that I was going home. 'You can't stop me going if I want to,' I declared.

Sylvia looked up and said, 'Now you know that isn't true, Veronica.' This made me even more furious. I went outside and literally banged my head against the wall.

I stayed outside until I could not stand it any longer. No one was discussing options; they were up to something and I wanted to know what. I marched into the office again and demanded to know what they were doing. I cannot remember what the answer was but it caused me to turn, go out and bang my head and fists against the whiteboard. I was aware of Sylvia asking me not to wipe off the writing. I turned and walked to the ward's exit door, which had been locked when the night staff came on, and leaned with my head and fists against it.

At this point someone came up and introduced himself as Dr Wilkinson, a registrar. He said that he was not really involved in my case but happened to be passing by. He suggested that we talk about things. I went with him and the SHO to an interview room. Like Julie, the registrar said that I had come to them that evening and must have realised that I needed help. He went on to say that I should be admitted to Wintle as there were no beds available at Phoenix. I stated once again that I was going home. Dr Wilkinson answered that they were concerned about my being alone and that I was not fit to go home, especially in the state I was in then. I persisted saying that I was going home. Dr Wilkinson then told me that I could go to Wintle voluntarily or under Section 3 of the Mental

Health Act. I replied that that was no choice. He replied that he was sorry but repeated that I was in no fit state to go home.

I went back to Phoenix and walked to and fro, getting even more agitated. I now had a nurse allocated to me, who stopped me whenever I went near the exit. Another nurse then approached me with a mixture of two drugs, which I took. This is not done simply to make behaviour manageable for the nurses; being so ruled by extreme agitation and frustration is not at all pleasant for the patient either. By the time that transport had arrived, the medication had taken effect and I had calmed down to some extent. When I arrived at Wintle, they showed me to a room. They gave me the same mixture of drugs, obviously not wanting to risk a return to irrational and awkward behaviour.

For someone who is normally logical in thought and would usually approach a controversial situation by having a rational discussion of the point at issue, my entire behaviour that evening was completely out of character. That is what being 'out of your mind' means. There are those who say that suicide is selfish, but selfishness has no meaning for someone whose mind is ruled by severe depression with its complete negation of your normal thinking ability.

Sometimes I would deliberately behave dangerously when I managed to leave the ward. After I had been admitted in June 1996, I left late one evening when it was becoming dark. Chris, a nursing assistant who later qualified as a psychiatric nurse, came after me. I walked to the village, but Chris blocked my way to prevent me going too far away from the hospital. On my way back, when it was quite dark, I walked in the middle of the road. Chris, who followed the usual hospital policy of not putting yourself in danger of becoming a second casualty, kept pace with me on the pavement. Drivers could hardly see me except when they were close, which caused them to suddenly slow down and go carefully around me. No doubt some of them knew that there was a mental health unit nearby and were not surprised at my eccentric behaviour.

There was another occasion when I spent several days in my car driving in the vicinity of Oxford. This was in January 1996. I was developing suicidal thoughts. I had stopped taking my medication. I was anxious and confused and my mood was going down. Nothing but black thoughts emerged from my hopelessness. I telephoned my GP, and Nick Rose at various times.

I told the GP that I did not want to go to the hospital, as it only made things worse. He said that my health was surely more important, to which I replied that my health was no good on its own.

I even telephoned Joy and told her that I would not be at my four o'clock appointment with Nick that afternoon, but would telephone at about a quarter past four. It was the only time that I have refused to attend an appointment with a consultant, GP or CPN. When I called Joy again, she told me that Nick was in his office with a patient. Since I refused to give my number (in a lay-by off the A40), she could not ring me back. She asked me to wait as she went to see what he wanted to do. She had gone before I could comment and was replaced on the telephone by Nick. I told him there was no point in getting better as things only got worse. I did not want to go into hospital – that also only made things worse. I wanted to be dead. Nick told me that he thought I was not in the right state of mind to take big decisions about whether I wanted to go on living or not. When I told him that my phonecard was running out, he replied that he did not know where I was but he would be in his office for the next three quarters of an hour, and advised me to come and see him.

I got back into the car. Quite impulsively, without consideration, I started the engine and drove to Littlemore. Parking at the front of the hospital, I walked in and around to Nick Rose's office. I knocked on Joy's door and almost immediately it was opened. Nick muttered a quick 'Oh' and I got the impression that for once in his life he did not know what to say. This was momentary and he got hold of the situation swiftly. He told me that he was glad that I had come. He offered me a cup of coffee, which I refused. He tried to reassure me that I had made the right decision but I was less convinced when he brought up the matter of admission. I said that I did not want to go into hospital but the answer was, 'Look, bear with me a minute while I go over and check the bed state.' As Nick got up he offered me a coffee again, which I again refused. He picked up a cup, filled it with cold water and, putting it beside me, said that he would leave me with that anyway. He must have deduced my dehydrated state from the sound of my voice. 'You really are not at all well,' he stated before going out.

I hardly had time to consider taking advantage of the situation when he was back with a Phoenix nurse, to take me to the ward. I twice refused to move and twice said that I did not want to be admitted. The second time, however, Nick answered, saying that he was sorry but I really must stay.

On admission I was, as usual, searched and anything considered dangerous was confiscated. A nurse looked through my handbag and took, among other things, a spare car indicator light bulb. A new nurse, Sue, took my keys. She confiscated my belts, a bottle of stain remover (what was that doing there?) and other such things, for which I was given a receipt. I was used to this. If I had my dressing gown they would take the cord, which always annoyed me.

They had even been known to search my visitors.

Nick came in briefly that Friday evening to once again tell me that I had made the right choice, though it seemed to me that it was not I who had made the decision.

I refused both drink and food and did not have the energy to rise from my bed or wash and change my clothes until Monday. Nick came in to see me on Tuesday afternoon. He took a chair and sat down. He explained that he was thinking of introducing a new antidepressant called venlafaxine, which he had mentioned previously. He also brought up the subject of ECT, telling me that it would have to be considered if I was significantly dehydrated, enough to cause physical problems, but I would have to bear with him on that one because it would be twenty-four hours before the results of my blood test of the previous afternoon would be known. He urged me to drink. 'We don't want you in the hospital on a drip,' he said, meaning the John Radcliffe Hospital, which was where I would have to go if I needed an infusion.

He returned a few hours later and questioned me closely on when I had stopped taking the phenelzine, as it was essential for it to be out of my system before I started the new drug. He decided to start it, but for safety I would have to be without treatment until the next Monday.

The second Friday I was there, I decided to leave. I was pursued by Simon, one of the new nurses, and a nursing assistant. Knowing that they would catch up with me, I deflected into an interview room near the exit, where I sat down with my face in my hands. Simon asked me to go back to the ward with them but I made no move to go. He must have decided that I was safe where I was if watched, so he asked Ellen, the nursing assistant, to stay with me. He left and returned quite quickly with a bleep for her, instructing her what to do if I made a move to leave. I knew that the bleeps had little pins which, if pulled out, set off the bleeps of all the other nurses in the hospital, with the result that nurses would descend upon you from all directions.

Ellen was later replaced by Jennifer, another nursing assistant. It must have been not much past six in the evening that I became aware of someone looking through the glass panel of the door, then entering the room. I looked up and realised that it was Nick Rose, presumably about to go home as he had his briefcase in hand. He must have called in at the ward before leaving, as he often did. Jennifer offered to leave but he told her that she was all right where she was.

In the ensuing conversation Nick sympathised with my unwillingness to be in hospital but said it was clear that I needed to be there.

He asked me how things were going, then remarked that it was unfortunate that I had to go without treatment for the first week but that it was necessary for safety. He acknowledged how difficult things were, as I was getting the worst of both worlds, since I was having withdrawal effects from the former drug without, as yet, any therapeutic effect from the new drug. I was still plagued by thoughts of self-destruction. 'I know it's tough,' he said in conclusion, 'but . . .' He warned me not to underestimate the way depression could colour all my thoughts.

It was after this that I finally relented and allowed Jennifer to escort me back to the ward.

A case conference was organised. During an earlier admission, a Newsnight team was on the ward as apparently Littlemore was the only place that arranged case conferences. Nick Rose had introduced them. Invitations were sent to the GP, the patient's family and the patient themselves. The named nurse, the relevant SHO and the consultant would also be present. They were usually organised when there was something of importance to be discussed or arranged, especially discharge. My conference happened to coincide with a visit from Katherine and Nicholas. The Saturday before the conference, Katherine had telephoned to arrange the visit. I therefore asked her if she would be at the conference with me and she said that she would if I thought it would be appropriate. I had pointed out in a letter to her and Nicholas that they represented one of my main supports and, as such, Katherine's presence would probably help.

During this time Tim Woodward was also very supportive, although he no longer worked at Phoenix. He gave me his office telephone number so that I could contact him if necessary.

It always helped to have a good GP who was easy to speak to. Nick Rose liked me to keep in touch with my GP and that certainly helped; the better they knew you the more easily they could judge the extent of your depression. One of my GPs, who was actually qualified in psychiatry, on my telling him that Nick wanted me to go into hospital, commented, 'Well, Dr Rose, like the rest of us, sees you suffering and knows that hospital is the best place to deal with it.' I was reminded of Dr Andrews and his reason for admitting me – 'You've suffered with this long enough.' The fact that major depression causes great suffering is not always taken into account by those who do not understand the reasons for your going into hospital.

While I was in London, I had a very sensitive GP, Dr Morrison, who appreciated how awful depression was. He was very easy to talk to. When he was due to be away for two weeks, he suggested that I make an appointment with his partner so that I would know him if I needed to see him during Dr Morrison's absence.

Dr Price, my present GP, has known me for over ten years. Continuity is sometimes a luxury, but it does help tremendously. This past summer, Nick Rose left after being my consultant for nineteen years. He knew me pretty well inside out by the end of that time. Apart from having very good personal traits for a psychiatrist, he was always supremely concerned about my being involved and informed. Tim Ackland once told me that he had asked Nick if I was to be included in my case conference. 'As far as I am concerned, Veronica's always been involved,' Nick 'snapped back', according to Tim, and Tim demonstrated the recoil that this response had caused. His typical hyperbole made me laugh. Tim could always cause me amusement if I was anywhere near appreciating it.

Nick usually gave me copies of reports and letters. Regarding the need to inform third parties, he was particularly circumspect. He once said to me that he was very careful about what he said to employers. He was always strict about confidentiality. There is absolutely no way that he would have spoken to Moira without my express permission. Dr Sanderson at High Wycombe appreciated this, for she was equally concerned about such matters. I have generally been impressed by OH departments I have dealt with.

Chapter 18

Moved from ward to ward – Time in Ashurst – Complaint to
Healthcare Commission

Naturally, not everything about Oxford was good and I had cause to
make complaints. Many beds were closed – too many in my opinion,
with unfortunate results.

In January 2005 I went out of hospital to stay overnight in my
flat. This was a usual part of discharge, which was organised gradually with the patient spending an increasing number of nights out
until he or she was ready for complete discharge. I came back on
the Friday morning, from my first night out, to be told that an emergency case had been given my room. I went and sat in the quad next
to Mia, a friend and fellow patient in the same position as me.

Eventually Mia was given a room on the ward, but there was still
nowhere for me. I began to feel distressed and angry. I wondered
why Mia should have the room and not me, then felt horribly selfish. Why shouldn't she have the room? I was still quite vulnerable
and was only at the beginning of the discharge procedure. I began
to feel distraught at the whole situation.

I was told that Nick Rose was still around and would come
and talk to me. This was my penultimate admission before he left.

I was seated outside the office when Chris came and invited me into the inner office. He said that there was one room, which was condemned, but could be made up with a bed. He was very apologetic and sympathetic.

It was while I was sitting outside the office, head in hands, that Nick came. He slid down the wall to sit on his heels next to me. He was fairly matter-of-fact about the situation. He told me that everything was being done to find me a bed but the situation was serious. At that moment, Chris was getting a bed to make up for me in one of the interview rooms until a proper room became free. Nick got up, said that he was off, and went through the double doors.

Chris and Emma made up the bed for me and found a bedside lamp. Chris remained very apologetic, and kept touching me gently to convey his sympathy. They left me, but Chris was soon back. He told me that a bed had been found for me, in Banbury. I could not quite believe it. They were sending me all the way to Banbury in the north of the county. Chris said that he would order a taxi to take me there and someone to accompany me. They were very nice to me in Banbury, although I remained unhappy about being in an unfamiliar ward. They told me that I would only be there until Monday, when they would return me to Oxford, so it seemed that I was to be there for the weekend.

Late the next morning, one of the staff came to tell me that I would be returning to Oxford; a taxi had been sent for and it would be there in about an hour. It seemed an expensive operation. My escort told me once again how bad they all felt about what had happened.

I was supposed to spend the Sunday, Sunday night, and Monday at the flat but, because of what had happened when I last went out, I didn't go. I drove out to the flat on the Monday morning, as I was due to see my CPN there at ten. Afterwards I returned to Phoenix.

Concerning the situation, Chris Moran wrote a long entry in my notes describing what had happened. At the end he wrote: 'It would be deeply regrettable if a similar debacle occurred on Monday and may cause an unacceptable degree of distress to Veronica.'

On the Wednesday, I had a meeting with Nick Rose and my CPN. I told Nick how upset I had been by having to be moved up to Banbury. He told me that more beds had been shut, something with which he disagreed. He had written a report in the *Psychiatric Bulletin*, on the subject of bed occupancy. There he referred to 'the most tenacious theme' being 'the bad effect of providing a service in the face of bed occupancy usually approaching 100%', which results in 'higher frequency of transferring patients between units than would otherwise be needed'. He recommended a bed occupancy of

85%. Last year, the Royal College of Psychiatrists named 85% as the target bed occupancy for all acute psychiatric units. Oxford was running at over 100%.

At that time, we were told to remove all our belongings from our room and take them home when we went on leave. Previously patients in Phoenix had left their things in their rooms, which was then locked while they were away.

On one occasion I was transferred to another ward, arriving in the evening. This was not the result of my having been on leave, for I wasn't near discharge. I was simply shown to a room and left. In the morning, a nurse leaned against the door jamb and said that I could make a cup of tea, then went away. I didn't know where to make a drink, apart from which, if they had bothered to assess my state of mind, they would have realised that I was too depressed to make a drink for myself. That morning the ward manager took me back to Phoenix in his car. I wrote to him afterwards complaining of the treatment, or rather the lack of it, that I had received on his ward. When he replied, he asked why I hadn't told him about it when I was in the car with him. He suggested that I may have been too angry. If his staff had done their job, they would have realised the profound state of depression I was in, causing me to be very withdrawn. Apparently it did not occur to the ward manager that I might have been too ill to feel like speaking. Did he assume that someone in a better state of mind had been sent to them?

I was in hospital from July 2004 to February 2005, a six-month admission. Given the length of the admission, and the fact that I had required sectioning, I think that more care should have been taken. However, I was actually moved around more than I had been before. First, I was sent from Phoenix at Littlemore to Wintle Ward, at the Warneford Hospital. I was not fit for discharge at that time but was moved on the grounds that I was the 'most settled' patient. I challenged that judgement. I have wondered whether my very withdrawn state led them to feel that I was 'settled' (whatever that meant) and less likely to complain. In recognition that I had been very distressed by the move, it was arranged for me to return to Littlemore, but to Ashurst Ward, not Phoenix. As far as I was concerned, this wasn't much better.

While I was there, I was moved from a single room to a double room, without any warning let alone any discussion of the change. The only time previously when it had been decided that I should go to a double room was some years earlier, in Phoenix. My named nurse was on duty but was not consulted. A nurse had come into my room and told me of the move. I was very distressed by this and, by the time she came back to give me a bag to put my things in,

I was crying helplessly. She ignored this, dropped the bag and went away. My named nurse came in at this point and asked me what I was upset about. When I explained, she said that my mental state would deteriorate if I had to share a room. She said that she would sort it out and I heard no more of it.

Normally I wouldn't object to sharing a room. Most nights during the coast-to-coast walk we had stayed in a youth hostel and I had shared a room with strangers and it had not bothered me. When I am depressed, however, I am much more vulnerable.

Having been told that in Ashurst I was to share a room, I became very distressed though this was ignored. I avoided the double room and spent a lot of time at the end of the corridor. I very much needed seclusion but had no room of my own to go to. I was eventually returned to Phoenix. Even after that, however, I was approached and told that I would be moved again. This time, I responded by leaving the ward and walking into the town centre. As usual when distressed, I walked and walked for miles. It was dark by the time I got to the city centre. The police found me and returned me to the ward. If I was so well and 'settled', why did they feel the need to call out the police as soon as I left the ward? Someone else was moved when they realised the distress it would cause me to be moved yet again.

When I was discharged, on 23 February 2005, I sent a letter of complaint to the Mental Health Trust chair, which was passed to the complaints manager. She asked me if I wanted the complaint to be treated as formal and I said that I did. All you got from an informal complaint was a letter of apology – sincere as this no doubt was, nothing was done, and I wanted something to be done about the position of patients being moved from ward to ward.

As part of the formal complaints procedure, there was an investigation by the Mental Health Trust. I received a letter from the chief executive in which she said that the manager of Vaughan Thomas Ward had made an investigation. I was not happy about this, since he had been the manager at Phoenix at the relevant time. Although I had every respect for him, I could not see that he was able to make an independent testimony in the circumstances. The report actually did little other than confirm the basic facts.

At the bottom of the letter, it said that if I wanted to take it further I could go to the Healthcare Commission. I decided to do this and wrote a letter describing the full circumstances. Although the chief executive had said in her letter that the position was not owing to financial matters, I expressed the view that finance, resulting in bed closures, was one of the obvious causes of having to move patients around. I did acknowledge that the Mental Health Trust had to contribute a large amount of money to the Oxfordshire Financial Recovery Plan, to save other hospitals in the county which had not, like the Mental Health Trust, balanced their books. As I pointed out, if there had been sufficient beds, I would not have had to be moved. I put forward the following points for consideration:

- a clear, written protocol should be drawn up which it would be obligatory to use whenever it was proposed that a patient be moved
- terms used should be objective and unequivocal
- a senior nurse and a doctor, preferably from the patient's team, should be consulted
- the patient should be interviewed (If they are unable to take a meaningful part in such a process, I would suggest that they are not in a fit state to be moved.)
- no patient should simply be presented with a *fait accompli* and moved
- the patient should be moved back to their own ward and, if at all possible, not moved a second time.

In my final paragraph, I attested that the care and concern I had received in Phoenix had been largely of a remarkable level and that the nurses themselves disliked the situation of having to move patients. I always feel obliged to acknowledge what is good.

My complaint was followed up to the stage where the Commission brought in an adviser, an expert in mental health care. A copy of my medical notes and any relevant letters had been obtained from the Mental Health Trust.

The final judgment was sent to me in a long letter from the case manager. Initially it set out the facts as I had put them in my original letter and recognised the points I had asked them to consider. It said that the adviser accepted that the moves were traumatic for me and was surprised that nursing staff had suggested that I was happy to move from Phoenix to Ashurst and was even looking forward to it. So was I. The adviser said that it was obvious from my complaint and my medical notes that 'these moves, and even proposed moves, had a detrimental effect on your recovery'. She noted that Nick Rose had visited me in Ashurst and had come to the same conclusion.

The letter said that in order 'to reduce or avoid transfers, trusts need to reduce their bed occupancy rates'.

The adviser 'suggested a number of steps that the Trust could take to improve the practices within the organisation'. She stated that:

- a written bed management protocol should be in place which included objective criteria based on relative clinical risk factors when identifying patients who can be moved at least risk to themselves

- the level within the organisation at which bed transfer decisions are made during 'office hours' and 'out of hours' should be explicit. This will often be the person acting in the 'bed manager' role
- there should be written information available, which informs patients that ward transfers may occur and that leave beds may be used if there are no alternatives available
- when a decision is taken to transfer a patient, this should be sensitively discussed with them and they should be supported to minimise the degree of trauma such a move may cause. A record of the reasons, the discussions and the patient's reaction should be recorded in the notes
- the trust should monitor the number of patients transferred for non-clinical reasons and the underlying reasons for such transfers with a view to reducing patient transfers.

The case manager at the Healthcare Commission said that he would contact the Mental Health Trust in writing and expected that they would contact me within twenty-five working days to tell me what steps they were taking in response to the recommendations made. He would ask the Mental Health Trust to copy any correspondence to him. He said that I could return to the Commission if I were not satisfied.

I subsequently received a letter from the Director of Nursing and Clinical Governance which detailed each recommendation and what was being done regarding them. I felt vindicated, as positive actions were being taken towards minimising the effects of transfers and they were going to be audited.

I must say that any complaint I have made to the Mental Health Trust has been dealt with very professionally. I have known people to be afraid of making a complaint in case it made a detrimental difference to their care. That certainly did not happen to me.

I would like to think that I am as ready to give praise as to criticise, as with my letter to Dr Rose in which I also referred to my appreciation of his secretary. After the time the two policemen stopped when I was in my car in the rarely used lane, and were very sympathetic, particularly the one who drove me back to Littlemore, I wrote to the chief constable of Oxfordshire and praised them for the way they had dealt with the situation. I went to the top so that their acts were recognised by their seniors, as I felt they deserved to be.

Chapter 19

Break-up of my relationship with Richard – Therapeutic relationship with Nick Rose – Move to flat in Littleworth – CPN from Thame – Solicitor's opinion

---

One thing that was finally settled was my relationship with Richard. I eventually decided to move my property from the house, as there seemed no point in leaving it there when I was not living there. My brother-in-law Keith hired a van and helped me to get my belongings.

Sometime after, I went to the house. Out of courtesy, since I was not living there, I did not use my key but rang the bell. The door was opened – by a young woman. She and I looked at each other, then I turned and walked rapidly away. I could hardly believe it.

So this was the explanation for his frequent absences while I was not only caring for his mother, but being heavily criticised by him for my lack of concern for her. What would his mother think of her dear son? She would no doubt have some excuse. It was, of course, the explanation for his infrequent visits while I was in hospital and his absence on the second night that I was home after my first admission. I remember Steve Johnson saying, 'This is indicative of something, Veronica' – indeed it was.

I was extremely distressed by this discovery. It made me feel so completely betrayed. How could he do this to me? – and as for that woman, I am afraid that my feelings about her were less than Christian. She was, I was sure, someone who worked with him and she would therefore have known that Richard had a partner. She must have seen me at his work social events. She knew full well about me. I really think that starting to go out with someone you know to be in a relationship is thoroughly despicable. Of course, it may be that Richard told her that our relationship was breaking up, but until she saw evidence of it she had no right to interfere.

I continued to meet Richard, but he did not break up the other relationship. I therefore told him that he would have to decide between us. When I first met him to find out what his decision was, he simply prevaricated. The second time, I told him clearly that I would make a decision if he did not.

'If you said you thought we could make it, I'd stay with you,' he said. What was that? A threat? A promise? As far as I was concerned, he was trying to make me take full responsibility for the relationship and that was something I was not prepared to do. I told him I took it as a no. It was the last time that I saw Richard, but I did get a letter from him in which he told me that he was 'settling down' – he could not even bring himself to tell me that he was getting married. I was devastated. For years I had felt humiliated by his evident view that I was not fit to marry – then he walked away with that woman and married her. I was very deeply hurt, in a way I could hardly express. I felt so deceived and distressed. It made me feel utterly worthless – Richard had betrayed me, showing little concern about it.

He did send me a substantial cheque, with no argument. The last few years had certainly brought out the worst in him but I had not stayed with him for ten years for nothing.

Following my withdrawal from our house, I lived in a series of different bed-sits, none of which worked out, until my cousin Jenny, as ever, came to my rescue and had me live with her. A little while later, Nick involved a social worker. I was not sure about this development. I had quite enough people involved in my care as it was. However, the social worker proved to be very helpful in getting me somewhere to live. Nick was prepared to write a letter to the effect that I needed my own accommodation for the good of my health. This was certainly true, as I discovered when I moved into the flat. Having somewhere to live of my own, even though rented, did wonders for my morale. Heather, the social worker, helped me to fill in forms and established that South Oxfordshire was obliged to accommodate me rather than Oxford city. I was therefore given a large one-bedroom flat in Littleworth, just next to the village of Wheatley. There were only six flats in the block and they were on a country road between two villages, Wheatley and Horspath.

Prior to finding this flat in Littleworth, I was offered a flat in Abingdon. Tim Woodward came to talk to me about it, as it was his community area and it was possible that I may be offered him as my CPN. Having discussed this, however, we decided that it would not be appropriate as it would interfere with our friendship, replacing it with a professional relationship that would not allow anything personal.

I moved into the Littleworth flat with nothing but a futon, a bedside lamp and a coffee table. There were no carpets on the floor or curtains at the windows. The church I went to in Thame came to my rescue when a friend put a notice up explaining the circumstances and asking for any unwanted furniture. Because I was not so well at the time, she gave her own telephone number so that she could sift out inappropriate offerings. As a result I received two single beds, a table that was just the right size for my sitting room, crockery and some table linen, all of which were really useful. Not a single person asked for any payment, but I wrote to each thanking them.

It caused some confusion, my living in Wheatley in the South Oxfordshire district. My CPN came from Thame in South Oxfordshire, but Nick Rose covered the Vale of the White Horse. In addition, Nick was my key worker at that time, a responsibility that usually devolved onto the CPN. Of course, I had been out of Nick's area from the beginning, having been admitted to Phoenix because there was no room in Wintle at the Warneford, the ward I should have been on. Nick simply kept me under his care, which was fine by me. Anyway, it sometimes took some explaining once a CPN from Thame was allocated to me.

I particularly trusted Nick because he always made every effort to ensure that I was properly informed about what was happening, either through telling me himself or copying letters to me. He always encouraged me to make my own decisions if at all possible, and to express how I felt. He was also very good at telling me if he thought that I had made a particular effort. I was used to people assuming that an admission to hospital showed weakness and lack of effort. On one occasion I was in hospital when Nick had a talk with me about how things were going. I felt that things had improved, to which he replied that he was sure that I had turned things around, adding 'you have – not me, not the team – it's you who have done it'.

Whenever I was discharged from the ward, I would leave a card for the nurses saying how much I appreciated their help. It did occur to me that I never actually told Nick how much I appreciated him. Doctors tended to be left out of such things. The doctor who had admitted me in Nick Rose's absence, when I was at GOS, had dealt with the situation very sensitively. I last spoke to him on the telephone when I asked him if I would see him again. He said that I would not. I therefore told him how helpful he had been and how much I appreciated his understanding. In return he thanked me, sounding very pleased and really quite surprised.

I wrote Nick a letter expressing my appreciation of what he did for me. At the end I wrote a paragraph saying how good his secretary, Joy, always was. She was not one of those secretaries who considered their chief role to be to stand between their boss and anyone who wanted them. Joy would always get Nick for me if convenient, or tell me when best to telephone back. If I was distressed, she would recognise it in my voice and make sure that she got Nick for me straight away. In the event I was glad that I had written in praise of her, as soon after he told me that Joy was retiring. I was glad that I had spontaneously written what I had felt when she knew that I was not writing simply because she was leaving.

Nick Rose was my consultant for a long time, during which he came to know me increasingly well. In a letter to my CPN he once said, 'although I felt she was fairly well, I thought I could pick up the early signs of strain' and in another letter, 'I have seen Veronica on a number of occasions in a rather similar state of mind, and at present feel it is most appropriate if she continue to try and work . . .' He knew me sufficiently well to be able to interpret any signs of problems.

In April 2007 I had a meeting with Nick and my CPN, Tim, in which Nick told me that he was leaving the NHS at the end of the summer. I had opened the meeting by telling him that my father had died a matter of days before. Nick therefore acknowledged that it was not the best time to tell me, but the news of his leaving was already getting around the hospital and he was concerned that I should not hear the news from anyone else.

Before he left, I asked Nick if I could see him on his own. The first thing he said to me when we were alone was, 'The depression is *not your fault*. It is *not your fault*.' He knew how plagued I was with guilt about my illness.

In 1995 I went to a solicitor for advice on a matter independent of SCBU, or so I thought. In explaining my position, and what had happened, I said something about the situation on SCBU and my reasons for leaving. The solicitor actually said that he was more interested in that, so I went into greater detail. He subsequently researched the events surrounding my leaving.

One of the aspects he looked into was the medical opinion of how far the work situation was to blame for my illness. He requested a report from Nick Rose, a copy of which was sent to me. Nick wrote of me:

> it also became clear that Miss Burton had a rather fragile self-confidence even when well; and a temperament characterised by worry-proneness, a tendency to be over-meticulous and a tendency to have fixed and fairly high expectations of herself and others . . . I would judge that disappointment at the re-grading significantly undermined Miss Burton's confidence at the time.

> This was particularly damaging in Miss Burton's case because of her double vulnerability of having low self-confidence lifelong, and having previously had a depression at the age of sixteen.

In conclusion, he stated:

> All I can say with certainty is that the re-grading profoundly undermined Miss Burton's sense of self-esteem, and this was an important contributing factor which predisposed her to the very severe depression she had developed by July 1989.

The solicitor continued his research and at the end came to the conclusion that I had good grounds for suing High Wycombe Hospital regarding my illness. One problem, however, was that we were well out of the three-year period inside which the case should have been pursued. However, it seemed that we could get around that by establishing that illness had prevented my pursuing the case any earlier. In the end, though, I decided against prosecution, as the solicitor advised me it would be a highly stressful business. I had no wish to make myself ill again over it. It did help me, however, to know that the case was worth pursuing – I had always agonised over whether it was all my fault, especially at those times when I was seriously willing to blame world disasters and the like on myself.

Chapter 20

It was soon demonstrated to me what prejudice against the mentally
ill really meant. There was, of course, Moira's description of me as
having 'mood swings', displaying 'rudeness and aggression' and
'lack of insight'. The archetypal madman. I am sure that she would
not have imagined that such descriptions of me would have been
accepted by anyone had I not spent time in a psychiatric hospital.
Then there was Moira's reason for not encouraging my colleagues
to speak to me directly, because I'd had a *mental* illness. (One has to
admire her courage in speaking to me alone – after all, I could have
strangled her. It's risky this speaking to mental cases.)

Mrs Newman had been careful to keep secret what was wrong
with me – not confidential but *secret*. She obviously felt that I was
very ill advised to put my name to an article about my illness. I,
however, have always made it a point of principle to put my name
to anything I write, although that has been hard at times, especially

in regard to that first article. I believe that if something is important enough for you to put it in print, then it is important enough to
own to. Not to do so colludes with the very people whose attitudes
you wish to oppose.

Once I was in hospital, I was dismayed at Richard's attitude.
When he came to see me, he was very apologetic about having to
explain to a work colleague, who took him to collect my car, why
it was parked at the Warneford. Even worse, when a close friend of
mine, Kathy, with whom I had started nurse training, telephoned
to have a chat with me, Richard tried to avoid telling her the truth.
Later she told me that he was 'very cagey' and made her so concerned that, had he not eventually told her the truth, she would have
driven from Derbyshire to Oxford to find out what was happening.
Knowing Kathy, I have no doubt that she would have done this.
It was amazing to me that he thought I would not like my own
friends to know that I was in hospital with depression. What sort
of friends did he think I had? What sort of friends did he have? My
friends have all been supportive and understanding throughout.
From what I later learned, however, his view of mental health and
mental hospitals was concurrent with that of at least 90% of the
population – full of stigma and prejudice.

I was once standing at the bus stop outside Littlemore Hospital.
There was a lady already there. She struck up a conversation with
me by asking me if I lived in the village. I said that I did not, but
rather that I came from the hospital. 'Oh, are you a nurse?' she
asked brightly.

'No,' I replied, 'I'm a patient.'

That proved to be a most effective conversation-stopper. The
lady looked at me suspiciously and took a few steps away. Well, I
suppose no one likes to risk being stabbed or strangled before their
bus arrives.

The fact is that a mentally ill person is appreciably more likely
(6% more likely, according to the Royal College of Psychiatrists in
2002) to be murdered than someone in the general population. In
1999 a report based on Home Office figures revealed that the number of homicides by the mentally disturbed had been falling steadily
since 1957, by 3% a year. In short, the mentally ill are more likely
to be murdered than to murder. This is directly counter to most
people's belief.

Nick Rose was asked whether he thought that my being in hospital, surrounded by ill people, did not make me worse. In all my
years of nursing, I have yet to hear anyone suggest that someone's
physical illness was made worse by their being with ill people in
hospital. The question seems to suggest that the worst problem my

179

illness presented was one of my simply being too impressionable. It is often thought that mental illness is a weakness best not encouraged by sympathy or compassion. Ignore it and it will go away. No one implied such things when I had meningitis. Of course, one of the difficulties with depression is that it can be a very serious illness, but it goes by a name that can be used to describe a temporary dissatisfaction. Most people are aware, if they think of it at all, that most people who commit suicide do so because they are depressed. Even that, however, can be regarded as a selfish indulgence.

My family often went on holiday in Cornwall, which is where my mother comes from and where we still have many relatives. One year, several of my family were staying in some cottages while Clare, Keith, baby Georgina and I went to join them. We camped on the local site. I slept under the awning, while Clare and Keith slept in the tent with Georgie in the camping cot.

That night I was horribly ill, repeatedly vomiting violently. By early in the morning, the vomiting seemed to have stopped. I had been sweating profusely so I decided to have a shower. The cubicles were within sight, so I walked slowly down. Once I got there, however, I felt awful and knew that I would not be able to stand in the shower; I therefore made my way back. I was getting near the tent and could see Keith, up early, outside the tent. I looked down and the grass went silver and the ground appeared to move around. I called Keith rather desperately and he got to me and grabbed me before I fell. He got me back to the tent where I collapsed onto the camp bed, gasping for breath. 'Vron, you've gone white!' Keith said.

Keith got me into the car and, having asked someone, discovered that there was a cottage hospital nearby. At the hospital, the receptionist was telling us to sit down when she looked up at me. She rushed off for a wheelchair. I saw a doctor, who was presumably a local GP. I was very worried as it had often been impressed upon me that I should keep myself well hydrated, otherwise my lithium levels would go up, possibly to dangerous levels. This naturally concerned me and, as I was in a state of shock, I kept mumbling about my lithium without really being aware of what I was saying.

They decided to keep me in overnight. The doctor took bloods and I, being rather more coherent by then, gave him my consultant's number and told him that Nick Rose would be able to tell him anything he needed to know.

This doctor said little to me and I had no reason to think that he did not believe me. Unknown to me, however, he decided that I had taken an overdose and that this was the explanation for my concern over my lithium levels. He told my family that I had taken an overdose, without saying anything to me. It was not until later that I discovered what he had said. He made no attempt to contact Nick, who would, I am sure, have told him that I would have done no such thing unless very seriously depressed, and would certainly not have joined a family holiday and then taken an overdose while basically well.

I was very angry with that doctor. He had no right to pass on his speculations to anyone else without my knowledge and permission. He said no such thing to me or I would immediately have put him right. I am convinced that he saw a young woman on psychiatric drugs and assumed that she was a serial overdoser. In not informing me of his absurd diagnosis, he was treating me like a child. Even medical personnel can stigmatise psychiatric patients.

Following my successful RSCN course, I should not have had trouble getting a job. However, I was refused at every interview I went to. I got in touch with the Royal College of Nursing (RCN) and one of their officers helped me. She thought it was peculiar herself. Although I had been ill, I was refused before they even referred me to OH so that cannot have been the reason for the refusals. The RCN officer suggested that it might be something to do with my references. She got a copy of one, which was fine, but took some time obtaining a copy of the other, from Maggie, a sister on the High Wycombe neonatal unit whom I trusted. She did so eventually, however:

> provided Veronica is not put under pressure, or in a stressful environment . . . after a period of sickness she was not able to cope well or under stressful situations, or under a lot of pressure . . .

I knew why I was not getting past the interview stage. I felt betrayed.

I remembered what Dr Sanderson had said in regard to Moira, that it was not for her to comment on my illness and that she should write a reference concerning how I had performed before my illness. Apart from the sister's actually writing it in a reference, she was wrong anyway. Even Moira had admitted to me that 'work has never been a source of stress to you'. In addition, we all need a certain amount of stress, but what is experienced by one person as a harmful stress is, to another, a helpful cause of an adrenaline drive essential for coping in an emergency. Once again, however, prejudice is at work in that anyone who has had a stress-related illness is assumed to be unable to cope with stress of any kind. Of the areas I most enjoyed, both neonatal care and paediatric accident and emergency are areas where an emergency may develop at any time. Confident that I knew what I was doing, I thrived on that uncertainty. All I needed was someone with some faith in me to trust me and to let me get on with my job. I had worked on paediatric accident and emergency as part of my RSCN course. When a critically ill baby was rushed to resuscitation, the staff nurse in charge gave me responsibility for him, knowing that I was a neonatal nurse. It took me and the doctor two hours to revive and stabilise the child, get essential X-rays and other necessary tests. By then, it was deemed safe to let another post-registration student to take over from me. I was going out of the door when the doctor called me back in order to thank me. The parents brought the baby to the department to see me when he was discharged, and it was lovely to see him when well.

I applied for a job at one hospital and received a letter from the OH doctor saying that she would want me to stay well for another year before she would pass me as fit. She admitted that this was despite my GP's and consultant's support for my return to nursing. I wondered why she had sought their opinion in the first place, since she obviously felt herself to know better than either of them. The letter finished *we do have extremely high standards*. The assumption was, presumably, that I could not reach them, although anyone who knew me acknowledged that I always worked to a high standard – too high, some felt.

I eventually got a job on the paediatric ward at the Nuffield Orthopaedic Centre, a specialist NHS hospital in Oxford. I was employed on a D grade, with the understanding that I would be given an E grade when it became available. Time went by and I was becoming impatient. The charge nurse who had employed me left.

One day I was in the nursing office when a staff nurse – who had only been qualified for eighteen months and had spent the whole time on the same ward – came in to be given congratulations. I asked what it was about and was told that she had been given an E grade. I could not believe it. Her only qualification was the RSCN and she was very inexperienced. Apparently the new charge nurse had advised her to apply when an E grade came up, despite knowing that I had been expecting an E for some time. She had not even mentioned it to me. When I told Nick about it, he commented, 'You've suffered a lot from prejudice.'

From the same ward I applied for a post working between the children's ward and theatre. My colleagues agreed that I was the ideal candidate. Several times I had been on night duty when theatre recovery had a child who had been in theatre for eight hours or more and needed intensive nursing care. Since none of the night theatre staff had the qualifications or experience to nurse the patient, I had gone down and looked after the child. Despite this, I did not get the post. My colleagues could not believe it, I seemed the ideal candidate.

Of course, you do not find prejudice in nursing alone; it is widespread in society. I had to cancel a holiday because I was admitted to hospital. I was not worried, as I was insured. It was then that I discovered that if your illness was psychiatric, you were not in fact covered by the insurance. There was no explanation for this exclusion. That would now, quite rightly, be illegal under the Disability Discrimination Act (1995), although life insurance policies can still make suicide an exception in the case of which they will pay out.

In May 1995 there was an article in the *Nursing Times* called 'Shadows of death'. The author referred to the open controversy about euthanasia, which caused patients to ask nurses to end their lives, and contrasted this to the lack of publicity given to the fact that nurses had been found to be the most likely of any female workers to end their own lives. The rate of suicides to normal deaths among nurses was nine times that of women doctors – the second most likely to commit suicide.

In response to this article, I wrote a letter to the *Nursing Times* but was somewhat dismayed when they printed it at full length, with the heading 'Depression worsened by prejudice from colleagues and managers' highlighted in yellow, as the lead letter. I wondered what my colleagues at the High Wycombe neonatal unit thought of it. I telephoned and found that actually they were in agreement with what I said. (I sought no comment from Moira.) As I wrote more letters, I became less concerned about how they were published. After all, I meant what I said. My original letter said:

> I read the article on suicide among female nurses ('Shadows of death', 12 April) with interest. The statistics suggest a connection between suicidal tendency and nurses' work. The issue of mental illness among nurses is central. If factors associated with work are significant, does it necessarily indicate nursing to be an inappropriate profession for people affected by mental illness?
>
> Prejudice within society is immense and other nurses, including managers, often share misguided beliefs which may damage an individual's personal credibility and professional future. It is believed that depression is evidence of inability to cope with the stress of nursing. The view that people with mental health problems should not be nurses is held by a large majority of the population (*Don't Fence Me In*, Radio Four, 18 April).

I have been admitted to hospital with suicidal depression and wrote an article about my experience. Before my admission I was recognised as a competent and capable staff nurse on a neonatal unit, confidently taking charge when rostered. Neonatal intensive care is thought of as particularly stressful, but coping with the stress of my job gave me the satisfaction of providing effective patient care. My job was not the reason for the unmanageable stress, but matters following the original grading exercise. I became deeply demoralised, filled with an ineffectual anger and a profound feeling of betrayal. It was these things that caused the emotional dysfunction that made it impossible for me to do my job. The grading implementation was for many a serious source of lowered morale. I summed up my feelings by saying, 'I feel as if I have been judged inferior to all those who I would previously have considered my peers'. To suggest that my depression proves me unsuitable for nursing confuses effect and cause.

Nurses affected by mental illness have to endure prejudice that sees it as inappropriate for them to have a responsible job. I lost my confidence through constant negative feedback which inevitably demoralised me. I suspect that it is matters peripheral to the performance of their duties that are creating unmanageable stress and making nurses feeling demoralised and unappreciated.

If a nurse becomes mentally unwell, to accuse her unjustly of being unable to take the stress of her job will simply compound the problem, intensifying loss of confidence and self-worth. Nurses are dedicated and caring people and the ability to provide for their patients' needs is of great importance. For the nurse recovering from mental illness, the prospect of returning to the profession that had given her purpose, self-esteem and a feeling of doing something of significance, may be her salvation and should never be taken away because of unthinking prejudice.

When my original article was published, some expressed surprise that I had put my name to it. Apart from considerations of honesty in the expression of opinion, anonymity simply colludes with attitudes one works towards removing.

The following two weeks saw the publication of two letters mentioning mine. One nurse, who had been in hospital for four weeks with suicidal depression, agreed that to return to nursing would indeed be his salvation. The other letter was from a nurse who found that the thing that left her 'deeply hurt and rejected' was the prejudice she suffered from her own profession. She said that because she was seeing a counsellor, she was seen as being 'extremely mentally deranged'. Unhappily, she felt obliged to resign her job. This letter was anonymous, which saddened me as I feel that part of protesting is being bold enough to give your name, rather than to act as if you are ashamed of the very thing you stand for. However, it is not for me to judge, I can understand only too well what makes people hide behind anonymity.

One letter that was signed and addressed to me came via the *Nursing Times*, with the staff having been asked to forward it. It was from Ian, a nurse from Aylesbury, who had suffered depression, although he was not hospitalised. The depression did, however, cause an anxiety attack that made him run from the ward he was working on. He then resigned. When he tried to take his resignation back the next day, management would not allow him to do it. He had read my letter and asked me 'if I wanted to take things further'. He and I met and decided that we would do what we could to advertise the problem of nurses suffering mental illness and their reception by their colleagues. So started a two-nurse campaign against prejudice and stigma. Ian was full of ideas about who to approach. We both sent letters to the press. I became the chief letter writer – when I became indignant about something, Ian would say, 'I feel a Veronica letter coming on.' We soon found that we had quite a high profile. The importance of what we were doing was revealed by a Nuffield Trust report that revealed that nurses suffered a higher rate of work-related mental illness than any comparable profession. A report published in 1995, from the Office of Censuses and Surveys, revealed – as already mentioned – that the ratio of suicide to normal deaths among nurses was nine times as high as among female doctors, the second most at-risk group. Also at that time a Mori poll revealed that, although the attitude of the public towards mental illness was improving, a large number of people still regarded the depressed as mad or mentally unstable. This report had been commissioned by the Defeat Depression Campaign. I was invited onto the committee of that campaign as a result of the work that Ian and I were involved in.

Ian and I called our campaign 'Stress in Nursing'. Tim pointed out to me that the acronym for this would be 'SIN'. I told him that that was deliberate, as indeed it was. The profile of this campaign was further raised when Ian and I were interviewed on the Channel Four programme *The Pulse*. I was featured on the main regional six o'clock news on Mental Health Day, at the request of MIND.

In 1997 the Pathfinder Mental Health Trust in London started to show a positive preference for considering applicants who had had mental health problems. They started to include on their employment advertisements a statement to the effect that they were 'actively seeking' people who had had such problems and that it would be seen as 'desirable' in an employee. In 2009 the Oxford Mental Health Trust is about to pursue such a policy, over ten years after Pathfinder. Better late than never, though.

One thing that came to light during the mid-1990s was the extent of bullying in the NHS. This was seen as an important cause of stress-related illness. At about the same time, people in all sorts of work areas began to sue their employers for stress-related problems originating in the workplace. The RCN reported that nurses might benefit from the case of a social worker who had two 'nervous breakdowns' (whatever they are) caused by overwork. He won £200 000 for loss of earnings. Nurses were, however, warned that winning such a case remained extremely difficult.

Of course, attitudes in the National Health Service reflected those within society. In 1996 the Samaritans produced research finding that more than one-third of the people surveyed considered that anyone who attempted suicide was only thinking of themselves. The same number believed that depressed people should 'pull themselves together' and that suicide was an easy way out.

The degree of stigma with which the public regard those with mental disturbance is undoubtedly due in large part to the attitude displayed by the media. In 2008 there was an effort to encourage reporters to take a more responsible attitude, and certainly not before time. It will be interesting to see the results of this undertaking.

In 1996 MIND published a survey on stigma, taboos and discrimination suffered by people with mental health problems, called *Not Just Sticks and Stones*.* I noticed three comments in particular:

- The most intolerant sector appeared to be the health and caring sector, with some of the worst cases of unfair discrimination in nursing and social work.
- 1 in 5 (20%) of the people who believed that they had been unfairly dismissed from their jobs were nurses, from other caring professions, or other NHS employees.

* Baker S, Read J. *Not Just Sticks and Stones*. London: MIND; 1996.

- There were reports of people being denied places on further education courses and professional training courses, particularly for nursing and other caring professions.

This endorsed the strong impression that Ian and I had already gained. The NHS was a particularly bad employer for those who had suffered mental illness, and nurses were particular targets.

After his precipitate resignation from Aylesbury, Ian never got employment with them again, despite sending in several applications. Instead he went to work at the bank (nursing agency run by the hospital) in mental health in Aylesbury, which resulted in his doing the RMN (Registered Mental Nurse) training. He also took a course in care of the elderly, an area in which there is a dearth of specialists. Despite that, he has not been employed for more than three years and tends to describe himself as an ex-nurse.

Chapter 21

Allitt case – Clothier report and its deleterious effect on prospects of nurses with psychiatric histories, or even those who have simply had counselling – Association with RCN Wing – Report *Mental Health and Employment in the NHS* – Ian goes north

---

Something that all nurses who suffered mental illness came up against at that time were the crimes of Beverley Allitt and their aftermath. During the months February to April 1991, the children's ward at Grantham and Kesteven General Hospital faced the sudden deaths of four children, and the unexplained collapse of nine other children and babies. Beverley Allitt, a nurse on the ward, was eventually charged with four murders, nine attempted murders and nine counts of grievous bodily harm on those same nine. She was given a life sentence for each charge. It was later decided that Allitt suffered from Munchausen's by proxy and she was sent to Rampton top-security mental hospital.

The Clothier report† into the events came out in 1994. I have read the report three times and the catalogue of failure on the part of almost all those involved still amazes me. Something that was picked up in the report and which was covered in one of its final recommendations was the fact that no one questioned why alarms failed to go off whenever a child collapsed with Allitt on duty. Of course, that realisation in itself would not have pointed to Allitt, as it would take sure evidence to convince one of the culpability of a colleague. However, it should at least have drawn attention to the fact that something was wrong. I cannot imagine why no one questioned the fact that alarms failed to go off, if nothing else was noted initially. The epilogue of the report asks why fragments of evidence that would have pointed to Allitt 'lay neglected or were missed altogether' and refers to 'a general lack in the qualities of leadership, energy and drive in all those most closely associated with the management of Ward Four'. The epilogue speaks of 'The ancient notion of the scapegoat' and warns against the urge to lay blame. One of the tragedies of the affair was the death by suicide of one of the night charge nurses on the ward. From what I read, it seems that she was one of the least to be blamed.

It would appear that, despite the Clothier report's warning against it, scapegoats were identified – they were the ordinary nurses throughout the profession who had suffered from psychiatric illness, those nurses whom Ian and I were seeking to defend and support. We received a letter from a nurse whose condition was likened to that of Beverley Allitt by OH, when it was declared that she was suffering from psychiatric illness.

I applied for one job and received a letter from the OH consultant saying that, despite the fact that both my GP and my consultant supported my return to nursing, she wanted me to remain in a stable state of health for at least another year before she would pass me as fit.

The Clothier report said:

> Any applicants with a history of absence through sickness, excessive use of counselling or medical facilities, or self-harming behaviour such as attempted suicide, self-laceration or eating disorder, should not be accepted for training until they have shown the ability to live without professional support and have been in stable employment for at least two years.

---

† Department of Health. *The Allitt Inquiry: report of the independent inquiry relating to the deaths and injuries on the children's ward at Grantham and Kesteven Hospital during the period February to April 1991.* London: HMSO; 1994.

This looked to me like an invitation for applicants to nursing to go without the care and support they needed. And what precisely is *excessive* use of counselling?

A mother wrote to the nursing press concerning her daughter, who wanted to be accepted on a nursing course. She had sustained a head injury in a motorcycle accident and suffered depression as a result. Her mother said that she refused to get the help she needed in case it compromised her nursing application.

There was also a letter in the nursing press from a nurse who 'had a defined mental illness' and was honest enough to admit to it on application forms – it took eighty applications before she was given an interview. She wrote that 'Allitt's despicable crimes . . . must not signal a witch hunt.'

Of course, the Allitt case was unbelievably horrific but, as the report states, ultimately Allitt herself must bear the responsibility for her appalling acts. The difficulty was that an over-zealous interpretation of the Clothier report was highly prejudicial to any nurse who had a mental illness history. This encouraged nurses to avoid being too honest about their medical history on OH forms, despite risking dismissal if it were discovered.

Our campaign went on for some four years, and stigma and prejudice kept presenting themselves. In 1997 it was suggested that nurses who appeared to be unwell should be reported to the nurses' disciplinary body, the United Kingdom Central Council (UKCC). The example given was of a nurse who continued to work despite being depressed, which, it was claimed, must have resulted in errors. They were, however, apparently unable to give any example of a mistake. I wrote in protest, to the *Nursing Standard*, giving my own experience when I had been admitted to a mental hospital as an emergency case when I had been at work only two days before. No one detected any errors made by me.

I said that nurses should counteract the assumption that mental illness and danger were synonymous, not perpetuate the idea. I did acknowledge that a nurse might be harmful, but that was extremely unlikely and nurses suffering mental illness had as much right as anyone else to be treated as individuals.

In August 1998 my local paper reported my case, with a photograph of me at my desk. Ian was in frequent contact with his local paper, which did an article on him.

Ian and I got in touch with Tom Sandford, the RCN mental health advisor. He was very sympathetic to our aims. Also within the RCN was the organisation for work-injured nurses (WING). Guinette Davis of WING was helpful, too. WING had previously concentrated on physical injuries but they were happy to have me on the council and taking a particular interest in mental health. I suggested that the council should interest itself in injuries that were not obtained at work but nevertheless affected the nurse's ability to work, or put her or him in need of particular help. I argued that there should always be a member of council with an interest in mental health, but this was not accepted.

In March 1999, at the RCN National Congress, Guinette and I found ourselves giving a seminar from which the original presenter had had to withdraw. There was a good write-up of the seminar in the *Nursing Times*, which quoted both Guinette and me. I pointed out that the Clothier Inquiry had failed to take any advice from psychiatrists or psychologists, relying on OH physicians who have limited knowledge of mental health problems. 'The Report produced a number of well-meaning recommendations that are nevertheless causing significant difficulties for many nurses with emotional difficulties who are seeking employment.' I said that problems for those with a history of mental health problems had existed before the Clothier report but acknowledged that its recommendations had worsened the situation.

It has to be accepted that Clothier was primarily concerned with the protection of the public, but their cause is not served by the refusal of employment to nurses whose experiences, in many cases, have served to increase their understanding of human suffering. This is the concept of the wounded healer, the idea that suffering can enhance one's ability to understand and care for others undergoing pain. It is true that nurses who have themselves endured ill health often have a greater appreciation of what patients are going through. We cannot benefit from this empathy if all nurses with any experience of mental illness are considered anathema.

In 2002 Carole Bannister, RCN occupational health adviser, sent me a copy of the report *Mental Health and Employment in the NHS*,[‡] which came to some important conclusions about the Clothier report. It said:

> The Clothier Report raised unreal expectations . . . A further outcome of the Clothier Report has been the stigmatisation of people who have experienced or are experiencing mental health problems.

It also said that OH physicians should get advice from mental health professionals, especially in complex cases. I certainly welcomed

---

‡ Department of Health. *Mental Health and Employment in the NHS*. London: DOH; 2002.

that after my experience of the OH doctor who refused to listen to the opinion of my GP and my consultant. The report, in many ways, vindicated what Ian and I were saying. *Mental Health and Employment in the NHS* stresses the need for careful risk assessment and acknowledges the effect of making people with mental health problems feel unable to reveal their history for fear of losing their jobs. It points out that this actively increases risk.

Ian and I wrote to anyone who might have an interest in the subject, from the Prime Minister and the Health Secretary down. One of the most helpful politicians proved to be the Prime Minister himself, the then much-maligned John Major. He took a real interest in what we were doing, and introduced us to other people who might prove helpful to us.

Many nurses withheld their identities and consequently wrote letters anonymously. The situation has improved but every anonymous writer bears witness to the fact that prejudice continues to exist.

Ian and I feel that one area where we helped was in the openness or anonymity dichotomy. We revealed our identities truthfully in every letter we wrote, even those that were published in the nursing press. In doing so, we helped to give a lead for other nurses and indeed more nurses wrote revealing their identity. Some attributed their doing so to the inspiration we had given. Our activities started long correspondences in the nursing press. They also highlighted the problem to unions, MPs and ministers and interested civil servants. We prompted Malcolm Rae, the mental health nursing officer, to introduce the subject to a relevant Department of Health working party. Malcolm Rae showed a great interest in our activities, and did what he could to help.

We have seen campaigns come and go, but prejudice is still out there. In January 2008, the 'Time to Change' campaign was launched; 'England's biggest ever mental health anti-discrimination campaign'.§ Will it solve the problem? We shall see.

It is often said that anyone can suffer from psychiatric illness. I suspect that there are people who will not, but you cannot prove a negative – no one can assume that they are immune from mental illness, certainly not through any belief that their character is too strong for such a weakness.

§ Campaign led by MIND and Rethink, evaluated by the Institute of Psychiatry.

Chapter 22 ▬

My present situation – The difference between feeling well
and feeling depressed

The longest I have spent out of hospital since 1989, when I was first
admitted, is two years and two months. So far it is one year and
ten months since I was last discharged. At present, I feel very well.
About a month ago I was speaking to Tim on the telephone and
remarked that I felt 'almost immune'.

'Immune,' he said, 'I don't like the sound of that word.' He soon
proved to be right. I went to Salisbury, forgetting my medication,
and went without it for several days. The result of that was that I
was not at all well for a couple of weeks after. On the Saturday,
I found myself feeling more down than I had for some time. Who
do you go to on a Saturday? When I was involved with Phoenix, I
would have telephoned the ward and spoken to one of the nurses,
but the wards had all changed. I had been in Allen only once, and
I did not consider myself to know any of the nurses well enough
to speak to.

The choice written down on the hospital's information was
the Samaritans, but my experience of them was variable. Besides,
I much preferred to talk to someone I knew.

The person I chose to contact was Mark Williams. Mark is our associate priest at St Mary's. He is also a professor of psychology, based at the Warneford Hospital. He was sympathetic and understanding. He spent some time on the telephone to me.

I am lucky to have Mark to refer to. It does occur to me that many people may be inclined to question my Christian beliefs in the light of what has happened to me through my life. It is certainly so that I have been plagued by a serious and highly disruptive illness. It has been the cause of interfering with my career such that I have by no means fulfilled the apparent promise that I displayed early on, before the depression returned. I would love to return to nursing, especially neonatal care, but I am very aware that many people would see my psychiatric history as being indicative of my inappropriateness for work in the area, though I would argue that it does not necessarily mean any such thing.

Because of my illness, I spent three years out of nursing. The result of that is that I will have to do a 'return to nursing' course, costing over £700, before I can be returned to the Nursing and Midwifery Council (NMC) register. I can only work as a professional nurse if I am on that register. Given that I am not sure whether I could once again be accepted for a nursing post, although I was accepted to work at the Nuffield Hospital (albeit I suffered from a significant degree of prejudice), it has to be questioned whether the course would represent a sensible investment. For my neonatal course at the John Radcliffe Hospital, I had to write a dissertation. I chose the subject of the neonatal nurse practitioner, at that time only an idea. Now there are many such nurses, and I would certainly have liked to achieve that position myself. Realistically, however, my career will never be on course again.

One of the major causes of my being subject to depression has been the fact that both of my parents have tended to suffer from depressive moods. For a period Mother had psychiatric problems, and Father was always subject to dark moods. I, however, seem to have inherited a double dose and my depression has been very serious. I do not actually believe that Christians are in any way immune from the world's ills; we suffer from such problems as much as anyone else. What I am aware of, though, is that whenever things have been at their worst, the right person has always been there for me. A prayer breakfast friend of mine commented, 'God always puts someone there – but it's up to you to find them.' Somehow, I have always been able to find that person.

When I was a teenager, I was very fortunate (if fortune is what you believe in), to have Pete Day recognise the seriousness of my problems, and give me invaluable support. Dr Hamber, my GP, was incredibly patient with me and extremely supportive. I do not know how I would have come through the experience without those two people; and, of course, Diana.

When I began to be depressed as an adult, Reverend Andrew Wilson was there. Not only did he provide a sympathetic ear, but crucially, he recognised the extent of my depression and the very real dangers it presented me with. He was willing to make that essential intervention when I was unable to express my own needs.

The registrar I saw in outpatients was responsible for me for only a short time, but he recognised the extent of what I was suffering and was compassionate and understanding. I do not know how I would have coped, insofar as I did cope, with my admission without the sensitive way in which he dealt with the situation.

Once I was in hospital, of course, Nick Rose became involved. I am sure that his contribution was essential in helping me through the whole awful experience. He always approached me with understanding, patience and compassion. When he left, someone commented to me, 'Dr Rose, very kind but –' But what? I wondered. But I would have been better off without kindness, understanding – what I needed was someone who would be firm with me, intolerant of my crazy obsessions, someone who would tell me to pull myself together and stop being so self-indulgent? All very well if you can dismiss depression as merely an indulgence. Nick had more faith in my determination to fight the illness than I did myself.

One thing I have noticed about feeling so well is that it is con-firmation of the difference between illness and being well. Along with being ill goes an immense feeling of guilt that 'I could be better if only I tried'. Part of being well is the discovery that I would never 'indulge' in feeling unwell if I had any choice. Serious depression is a deeply painful experience, one that causes you to feel that you would literally be better dead. There is no way one would make a choice to be in hospital in such a state. I am only too glad to be free of that awful state and hope that its absence continues.

Depression is not an illness that can be cured. The best that can be hoped is that it can be controlled with various treatments until it spontaneously goes into remission. My depression was seen as treatment resistant for a long time, because no drugs could be found to effectively treat it. The MAOIs and lithium that I am now on proved most effective, though even that combination has not been completely successful. We must assume that my present state is explained by a spontaneous remission.

Postscript

As Veronica's psychiatrist, I have been invited to add a postscript. A reflection on her words, read for the first time yesterday. Words that at times show such transparency and rawness that I was stopped in my tracks. For someone to be so eloquent in describing moments of virtual inaccessibility is like stumbling on a secret room in a familiar building. And to have that given as a narrative over a period of over 20 years contact with someone is a real gift.

So, what are my reflections? Well, most humbling is the reminder of the way fleeting gestures or phrases can resonate years later. None of us knows how 'what we say or do' is experienced by others. We have no control over this. And yet Veronica's account bears witness to how exquisitely sensitive she was to what was going on around her, and the lasting importance of certain words or actions. Indeed, the sensitivity of her antennae and the busyness of her inner world all seemed to be in overdrive at just the time she appeared closed down. The sheer amount of thinking involved in working out what was going on, who could be trusted, what this or that really meant. As a reader I felt the claustrophobia of her situation, the exhaustion of her trying to deal with yet further recurrences of illness. And the contradictions thrown up in her relationships with those caring for her. In illuminating these previously inaccessible corners of her illness experience, she forces me to challenge my own taken-for-granted version of her history. Familiar territory seen from another perspective suddenly seems perturbing.

Most important in this re-evaluation is the way Veronica's life emerges as a full story. Not just of a fight against illness, but a journey of whimsical childhood memories, shifting family relationships, and hopes and disappointments. A much richer world than can be captured in the psychiatric interview. It sounds morbid, but on the occasions I have attended a patient's funeral, I have always been moved by the glimpse I am given into the other life of that person, the side of them that is too often hidden from view, revealed in the recollections of mourners. As psychiatrists, too often we are drawn into seeing people through a lens of illness, as if this was their only identity.

Veronica's constant dilemma was navigating the difficult edge of both being a nurse, and needing to be nursed. And of at times feeling she was a failed nurse, helped by others who were not failing. The flip needed to achieve this role reversal is not easy, but I think Veronica manages to connect these two worlds very effectively through her advocacy for nurses who have experienced discrimination at work because of mental health problems. She is all too aware of the shadow that prejudice can cast over a health professional's career.

This in a way brings me to reflect on the invisible way power quietly but rather menacingly haunts Veronica's account. In the sense that she is embraced by the instruments of power. The labelling process of doctors, the use of hospital wards as safe places, the legal apparatus that can constrain a person's liberty (although not their rights). All this machinery of state, the result of centuries of discourse about the 'mentally disordered', bearing down on the needs of one emotionally naked individual.

For Veronica, this 'machinery' seemed both a source of security, where retaining a sense of control and autonomy could be negotiated, as well as a focus for small acts of rebellion. And for me, as an agent of the machine, the most important therapeutic value was the fostering of trust. However, the interplay between the power of the machine, and the trust held by a vulnerable individual was to be severely tested by two recurrent events in Veronica's illness. The possibility of having ECT; and the prospect of being detained in hospital under the Mental Health Act.

I hadn't realised it at the time, but clearly for Veronica, any talk about ECT was experienced as an act of terror in a world that at times seemed to be Kafkaesque. And when everyone seemed to be in on it, all persuading her of ECT, the fear and sense of being the victim of a conspiracy is palpable. Such are the unintended consequences of trying to do the best. But clearly there are lessons to learn from Veronica's account. That perhaps such conversations about treatment need to be more contained. But I was moved to hear that Veronica, even at her most non-communicative, felt that she could influence events, and retain some degree of control. For me, that is the most important thing. For to assume that, as a professional, you always know best, risks trampling on the last threads of selfhood that Veronica was quietly struggling to hang onto. I felt that by supporting her to take judgement calls, even as she was on the edge of losing the capacity to take decisions, was a way of trusting her. And as she herself points out, being trusted by others is an important part of restoring and maintaining identity and self-respect.

And the Mental Health Act? I shrank in horror at the way Veronica experienced this as coercion, against all my principles of fostering free choice. But in truth, the Mental Health Act is always there, a backstage presence, with a power that can invoke a dark mythology in the minds of patients who converse on our wards. It is the tooth and claw of the machine, albeit with beneficent intent (although this is not true of all cultures). And achieving that balance between respecting someone's autonomy, and yet sometimes having to take over decision making is never easy. For a patient, knowing that the consequences of saying no could result in a Mental Health Act assessment can feel intimidating. For as much as it is sensitively explained as the natural consequence of decisions made by the patient, it may be heard as a threat, a form of arm-twisting to do what the doctor wants. So it is informative for psychiatrists to hear Veronica's voice on this.

I suppose finally I am left feeling enormous admiration for an individual who has struggled for so long to master such a malignant depressive disease, yet who has retained hope, and kept open a future for herself. She has always fought to maintain control, never finally submitting to the slavery of illness. And the most recent evidence of this is her tenacity and feistiness in taking a stand on behalf of those working in the health field who experience prejudice when they develop mental health problems. We are all tested in different ways, but to be tested by recurrent severe depression is a burden of a particularly invasive kind. To repeatedly survive it and furthermore to benefit others by taking a stand requires considerable courage.

Nick Rose
Oxford
November 2009

List of acronyms

I am afraid anything that touches on nursing or medicine includes acronyms. Here is a list of those that appear in the book.

CBT   cognitive behavioural therapy
CPAP   continuous positive pressure ventilation
CPN   community psychiatric nurse
ECG   electrocardiogram
ECT   electro-convulsive therapy
GOS   Great Ormond Street Hospital, London
IPPV   intermittent positive-pressure ventilation
IVF   in-vitro fertilisation
JR   John Radcliffe Hospital, Oxford
MAOI   mono-amine oxidase inhibitor
NMC   Nursing and Midwifery Council
OH   occupational health
pCO^2 partial pressure of carbon dioxide (Boyle's Law)
pO_2 partial pressure of oxygen
RCN   Royal College of Nursing
RSCN   Registered Sick Children's Nursing
SCBU   special care baby unit
SHO   senior house officer
TTO   to take out
UKCC   United Kingdom Central Council (now superseded by the NMC)
WING   Work Injured Nurses' Association

Glossary

Amitriptilyne (AMT) The first antidepressants with real effect were the MAOI's (see below), but they had the disadvantage of requiring a carefully observed diet. Until the advent of alternatives, the tricyclics, of which AMT is one, were drugs of first choice for depression. I was treated with tricyclics during my teenage years, in the seventies, and as initial drug therapy in Phoenix.

Beck Inventory A multiple-choice type questionnaire for the use of psychiatrists, psychologists and allied professionals, that seeks to demonstrate clinical depression and indicate the degree of signs and symptoms suffered by the person completing it. There are other questionnaires used for similar reasons. The Beck Inventory was the one I became most familiar with, as I was most often given that one to complete.

Chlorpromazine (CPZ) A phenophiozine, used in psychiatry as an anti-psychotic. It also has an hypnotic effect, hence I was mainly given it to allow me to sleep. Given in smaller doses, during the day, it had a calming effect and helped to control excessive anxiety.

Community Psychiatric Nurse (CPN) I initially had to change my CPN quite a few times, but I found each one helpful and supportive. For a great part of the time I have been visited by my CPN on a weekly basis. I would very likely have had to spend more time in hospital if I had not had that vital support in the community.

Constant positive airways pressure (CPAP) A ventilator is a machine which breathes for the patient. The newborn has particular needs for ventilation, apart from those of infants or anyone older. CPAP is often used to 'wean' the baby off the ventilator. It maintains a continuous, low level of pressure which has the effect of keeping the airways open while the child breathes out. Inspiring air against the pressure of collapsed airways would be too much of an effort for the baby and result in respiratory collapse.

Data Sheet Compendium Each drug has a data sheet containing essential information for the professionals prescribing or administering it. These always contain advice on therapeutic dosage. Some include information about the amount that will cause dangerous overdosage. The Data Sheet Compendium contains a copy of each of these information sheets.

Electrocardiograph A test which produces a graph corresponding to the electrical activity of the heart.

Electro-convulsive therapy (ECT) A treatment that can be highly effective in relieving severe depressive symptoms. ECT is delivered while the patient is under anaesthetic, and a muscle relaxant avoids any trauma caused by muscle contraction during the induced fit. Without an actual fit occurring the treatment does not have any therapeutic effect. Some patients complain of serious side effects and would like to see the treatment banned, though others see it as the only treatment that is really affective against their depression.

Groups A group consists of patients, and perhaps one or two staff. A well-run group can be helpful and supportive for patients. Patients are encouraged to help each other within the group. In the therapeutic community, groups are extensively used, including the community meeting, to which all staff and patients are expected to go. The dynamics of the group may need particularly careful handling on some occasions.

The Healthcare Commission An independent body that inspected hospitals and their services. It reviewed complaints from patients in the NHS. It was superseded on 1 April 2009 by the Quality Care Commission, which combines the Healthcare Commission, Commission for Independent Health Inspection and the Mental Health Commission.

Intermittent positive pressure ventilation (IPPV) Term describing action of a ventilator when the baby is relying entirely on the machine to breathe for him/her.

Lithium Essentially a mood stabiliser, lithium is used in various states of depression. The main problem is that the patient must avoid becoming dehydrated, as this could have serious consequences. Fluctuations in sodium levels can also affect lithium levels.

Mono-amine oxidase inhibitors (MOAI) Can be very effective, but tend to be a last resort because of the possibility of dangerous interactions with certain popular foods such as yeast extracts (Oxo, Marmite, Bovril), hung game, processed meat, red wine (especially Chianti) and cheese. There is also a list of drugs that cannot be taken concomitantly.

Munchausen's by proxy Munchausen's is a condition where the sufferer fabricates illness in themselves. The 'by proxy' disorder is Munchausen's in which the fabricated illness is inflicted on another. Sometimes it can result in a person afflicting extreme harm on another in an effort to convince professionals of the genuine nature of the illness/condition. It can be a mother abusing her child or, as in the Allitt case, a carer causing harm.

Paediatric intensive treatment unit (Paed. ITU) Once a baby is discharged from SCBU he/she is never re-admitted, because of the risk of infection. If re-admission is necessary, the child will be taken to a children's ward or paediatric ITU, depending on need.

Partial pressures pO_2/pCO_2 In a mixture of gases, each gas exerts a pressure directly related to its amount within the mixture. (The description of which some chap called Boyle was first responsible, I believe – no doubt his description was somewhat more elegant than mine.) In short, oxygen and carbon dioxide each exert a partial pressure. To get a usable and accurate reading of blood gases requires a sample of arterial blood. The kindest and most efficient way to do this is by the use of a catheter inserted into the umbilical artery. It was pO_2 that was first measured transcutaneously, but this measurement was more problematic in the case of pCO_2. These difficulties have fortunately been overcome. Transcutaneous measurements are reasonably reliable but they need to be compared to an arterial sample at suitable intervals.

Section (of the Mental Health Act) In psychiatry the word 'section' usually refers to sections of the Mental Health Act 1986, which allow qualified personnel to take on certain powers in the interests of a patient who is unable to act beneficially for themselves owing to mental disturbance. The need for taking on such legal powers needs to be agreed as appropriate by two people qualified under the Act, who do not know the patient. This is usually another doctor and an approved social worker. Changes made in the Mental Health Act 2007 allow psychiatric nurses to qualify as approved personnel in this situation. A section may affect the patient's rights to refuse admission, leave hospital or refuse treatment. Use of a section requires a careful observance of safeguards, to ensure that all actions taken are in the patient's best interests.